"The perfect book for parents who feel ill at ease
or ill-equipped to discuss sex with their kids."
—*USA Weekend*

HOW TO TALK
WITH TEENS ABOUT LOVE,
RELATIONSHIPS,
& S-E-X

A Guide for Parents

HOW TO TALK
WITH TEENS ABOUT LOVE,
RELATIONSHIPS,
& S-E-X

A Guide for Parents

AMY G. MIRON, M.S., and CHARLES D. MIRON, Ph.D.

free spirit
PUBLiSHiNG®

Helping kids
help themselves™
since 1983

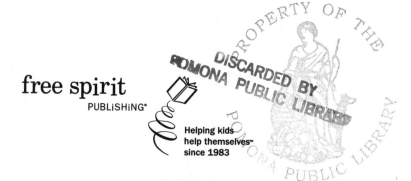

Library of Congress Cataloging-in-Publication Data
Miron, Amy G., 1947–
    How to talk with teens about love, relationships & S-E-X ; a guide for parents / by Amy G. Miron and Charles D. Miron.
        p.   cm.
    Includes bibliographical references and index.
    ISBN 1-57542-102-X
        1. Sex instruction for teenagers. 2. Parent and teenager. I. Miron, Charles D., 1944– II. Title.

HQ35 .M592 2002
649'.125—dc21
                                                                    2001040906

Author photo by Jeannie Harrison

10   9   8   7   6   5   4
Printed in the United States of America

Free Spirit Publishing Inc.
217 Fifth Avenue North, Suite 200
Minneapolis, MN 55401-1299
(612) 338-2068
help4kids@freespirit.com
www.freespirit.com

Dedication

This book is dedicated to our daughters, Jill and Lynne, who have been our constant source of joy. We are so proud of the people you have grown to be. Thanks for making our world a better place. We are truly blessed.

Acknowledgments

We'd like to thank the many clients and students who over the years have shared their lives with us and allowed us to learn from their pain and their victories. Thanks to Mitch, who got us to Marilyn, who got us on our way. A special thanks to all of our teachers over the years, especially William Masters and Virginia Johnson, who started our professional journey.

Thanks to Rabbi Bruce Lustig for his love of kids and families and for his courage to be on the cutting edge with us. To the CCBC research librarians who were always willing to find our articles—mainstream and obscure. And we're grateful for Mugs, who rescued us on that awful Sunday morning when we lost our toolbar. Thanks to Fran for generously sharing her creativity, even with tired feet.

Our hearty thanks to the entire Free Spirit staff—a more wonderful, cheery, competent bunch of people couldn't be found. A special thanks to Amy B., who kept us straight; Jennifer, whose research skills kept us current; Margie, whose insight, strength, and kindness we greatly appreciate; Sid, who pulled it all together; and Pamela, who will always have our gratitude. And what can we say about Yvette, except that we were blessed to have an editor as sensitive to our voice. Her warmth, humor, and patience made the sometimes painful process bearable.

And most of all, our heartfelt thanks to Judy Galbraith, who encourages the free spirit in all. Her steady hand at the helm has helped at each step on the way. May the winds be kind to her and always take her where she wants to go.

CONTENTS

INTRODUCTION

"What's a woodie?" your thirteen-year-old asks.

You feel a twinge in the pit of your stomach. You know an answer like "Woody? Oh, Woody Allen! He's a famous movie director!" isn't going to cut it. You can't put it off any longer: The time has come to talk with your teen about love, relationships, and S-E-X.

You're faced with the dilemma most parents face: You want your teen to have a happy, well-adjusted sex life . . . as an adult. You'd prefer that he* not make the same mistakes you may have made when you were younger—as a result of being ignorant or misguided, or perhaps because the adults in your life were too reserved or embarrassed to talk with you openly and honestly. If you learned about sex the hard way, you want to make it easier for your child. You hope that the sexual values and standards he adopts will be similar to your own, and you'd like to be able to sit down and talk about issues like sexually transmitted infections (STIs),** teen pregnancy, the value of waiting, and the power and wonder of love. But you may not have much information on some of those topics, or you may have information but not know how to share it with your child.

And you worry. What if you're planting ideas in your child's innocent mind? By giving him information, are you also giving him permission to be sexually active? In the parent workshops we run, this is a common concern. But study after study (and our own experience) shows that sexuality education *does not* encourage teens to start having sex. It *does not* increase the number of sexual partners a teen might have, nor does it increase the frequency of intercourse. In fact, studies consistently show that good things happen when teenagers are educated about sexuality—and that the price of sexual ignorance is dangerously high.

The United States, which has one of the highest teen pregnancy rates of any developed country, could learn from other nations. For many years, the government of the Netherlands has openly given out information about sexual issues through television, radio, and magazines. Sweden has had a compulsory sex education program in its schools since 1956. The teen pregnancy rates in these countries are among the lowest in the world.[1] In the United States, one study found that inner-city girls who participated in a school-based pregnancy prevention program had fewer pregnancies and postponed

---

* Throughout this book, we alternate the use of *he* and *she*. We feel this is less awkward and much easier to read than repeating "he or she" and "his or her." Except for chapters or statements that refer specifically to boys or girls, the information provided applies to both.

** Throughout this book, we use the phrase "sexually transmitted infections" (STIs) instead of "sexually transmitted diseases" (STDs). This is in keeping with language used by the World Health Organization and Planned Parenthood, among others.

first intercourse longer than girls who didn't take part in the program.[2] So you can relax. When you provide your children with sexual information, you're not giving them ideas or permission. It's far more likely that you're helping them be sexually responsible.

JUST THE FACTS

■ When adults and teens talk about sexuality, teens are more likely to delay first intercourse or to use contraceptives if they are sexually active.[3] According to one study, young adults reported wishing their parents had shared more information with them about sexuality.[4]

■ Each year, almost one million teenage girls become pregnant.[5] While teen pregnancy and birth rates are declining, four out of every ten girls in the United States still get pregnant at least once before age twenty.[6]

■ Each year, there are about four million new cases of STIs among teens.[7] About one out of every four sexually active teens will become infected, and most will be girls.[8]

We know it's hard for many parents to talk with teens about love, relationships, and sex. Part of the problem is that it's difficult for parents to imagine that their children are sexually aware, even more daunting to think they might be sexually active. They're so young—what's the big hurry?

JUST THE FACTS

■ Most young people in the United States start having sexual intercourse in their middle to late teens. More than half of all seventeen-year-olds have had intercourse.[9]

■ In 1999, over 8 percent of students reported having had sexual intercourse before age thirteen.[10]

■ Some teens are having oral sex as early as middle school. Most aren't aware that they can get STIs from sexual behaviors that don't involve intercourse.[11]

The reality is that your kids probably know a lot more about sex than you think. They're children of the Information Age, adept at surfing the Internet and cable channels, handy with VCRs and DVDs. Information (and misinformation) about sex is everywhere. Even if your teen is not on the computer, if she's watching TV she's bombarded with sexual content—and sexual practices that are unsafe 89 percent of the time.[12]

Graphic sexual activity, once relegated to pornographic movies in grimy theaters, is now the norm for mainstream films. The rating system devised to keep underage kids out of R- or X-rated films has been rendered virtually useless by the technology found in many homes and by apathetic theater owners. If your kids aren't allowed to watch certain movies at your house, chances are they know someone whose parent is less vigilant—or they have a friend who can download them from the Internet. *The real choice you face as a parent is not whether your kids will get a sex education, but how they will get it, what it will include, and who will do the teaching.*

Not long ago, a sixteen-year-old girl we'll call Lindsay made an appointment with us. When she sat down to talk about her concerns, she was obviously embarrassed. Finally, after much hesitation on her part and encouragement from us, she managed to tell us what the trouble was: She thought she might be frigid.

Lindsay and her friends had parents whose jobs required them to travel often. During these absences, the teens were left with little or no supervision and got into the habit of throwing parties. Drugs and alcohol were readily available, and the favorite party game was casual sex.

The person hosting the party would use the master bedroom, awarding the other bedrooms to close friends. Everyone else bedded down in the den or living room—wherever there was space. It wasn't unusual for more than one couple to be in the same room.

Lindsay was uncomfortable with this behavior. Try as she might, she couldn't put aside her feeling that it was wrong. Despite peer pressure and ridicule, she had not been able to join in. She was still a virgin. She sought our help because she thought there might be something wrong with her.

Lindsay's dilemma may be extreme, but tells us a great deal about the problems teens face today. Through the media and in real life, they're bombarded with expectations and images about sex and intimacy that are in conflict with what their parents believe is right (and often with what they themselves believe is right, since many teens, like Lindsay, aren't sexually active). They're told to wait until marriage to have sex, but they read about single movie stars and rock stars having children. They see TV shows and movies that glamorize casual, unprotected sex, often in conjunction with drinking and drug use.

When it comes to the broad issues of human sexuality—love, intimate relationships, sexual values, sexual choices, respect for one's body, respect for others, sexually responsible behaviors, assertiveness—many teens are offered little education or guidance. They often lack the basic information they need to make positive, healthy decisions about sexual behavior, yet they're making those decisions at younger ages.

JUST THE FACTS

Fifty-three percent of teens say the main reason they don't use contraception is because they're under the influence of drugs or alcohol at the time.[13]

You can't assume that sex and family life education classes in school will give your teens the information they need. Many sex education classes are little more than anatomy lessons, focusing primarily on reproductive issues. At best, they alert perceptive teens to the dangers of unprotected sex, though our experience with young teens has not shown this to be the case. At worst, they lull parents into a false sense of security that their children's sexuality education is being taken care of by the school board.

But it's not. More than ever, parents need to take an active role in their children's sexuality education. In the United States, federal pressure is pushing the public schools toward abstinence-only sex education. In most of these programs, acceptable sexual behavior is summed up in one word: DON'T! This means that many teens will not be given information in school about birth control or how to protect themselves from STIs.

In short, today's sexual landscape is a minefield. Allowing our teens to wander in continued sexual ignorance is simply unacceptable. As concerned parents, we need to educate ourselves so we can help guide and protect our children.

About This Book

Teens need to understand the whys and hows of social and sexual behavior. They need to develop standards and skills that will enable them to do what they believe is right in the face of opposing pressure. When the time comes for them to decide to be sexually expressive, they need a basic understanding of relationships, love, and sexual pleasure—and the potential emotional and physical consequences.

We feel it's critical for parents to present the issues of sexuality and relationships within the context of a value system—a way for teens to make sense of the confusing and contradictory messages they may receive. Obviously, that value system will differ from family to family. We won't presume to tell you what your values should be. But we can help you clarify what they are and suggest effective ways to communicate them to your teen.

Much of the time, teenagers act independently in the world. They make their own decisions about relationships and sex. As parents, we can guide our children and let them know what our values and beliefs are. We can tell them what we want and hope for them. But we can't control what they do, which makes it all the more important to give them real information about sexuality and put it in a context that helps them understand it.

We wrote this book to help you:

- overcome any discomfort you may have about dealing with sexual topics
- clarify your values and beliefs about sexuality and relationships
- gain more knowledge about sexuality and intimate relationships
- understand teens and their world
- understand the decisions teens face about relationships and sexuality
- develop a customized program of sexuality education—as a process, not a one-time event
- learn ways to communicate effectively with your teen
- identify abusive relationships and harassment and learn ways to deal with them
- create a forum where you and your teen can talk, raise concerns, and find answers about sexuality

A brief aside before we continue: Every family is unique. Each family member is unique. Just as we won't assume that you're heterosexual, we respectfully suggest that you not make that assumption about your teen. Consider, for example, that somewhere between two and twelve percent of all people are gay, lesbian, or bisexual.[14] Parents need to personalize their sexuality education program to each child's needs, whatever those needs may be. This book can help you do that.

How to Use This Book

How to Talk with Teens About Love, Relationships, & S-E-X is divided into two main parts. Each part includes "Try This" exercises, questions to think about, suggestions for things you might say to your teen, "What to Say?" sample dialogues, "Just the Facts" boxes, and real-life examples.

"Part I: Steps on the Way to Talking with Your Teen" takes you through a series of steps that will help you create and implement a strategy for your teen's sexuality education. You'll examine and clarify your values, determine your goals, gain a greater understanding of your teen and teen relationships in general, develop a model of sexual behavior appropriate for your teen, and learn ways to communicate more effectively.

We hope you'll have many "small" conversations with your teen. The more you talk with each other about love, relationships, peer pressure, choices, the emphasis placed on sex by the media, and so on, the more comfortable you'll both feel when you sit down to talk about specific sexual content. In the first five steps, you'll find several ideas for topics to discuss with your teen. Step 6 shows you how to make the most out of communicating with your teen.

"Part II: Issues to Know About and Talk About" presents current, factual information on a full range of sexuality and relationship issues. What you choose to share will depend on your teen and on your values. Within each of the issues, some parents will want to share all of the information. Others will want to share some of it—or none of it. Our goal is to provide you with as much information as we can to prepare you and your teen for almost any situation that may arise.

Maybe you've already started talking with your children about sexuality. Maybe you haven't. Or perhaps you feel that your attempts to do so have been awkward and unsatisfactory. We'll suggest ways to broach the subject naturally and correct any misinformation you may have inadvertently given your child in the past.

The "Try This" exercises are meant to be interesting and even fun. Most require nothing more than paper, something to write with, and a lively imagination. We hope you'll use them as icebreakers and springboards to discussion about sexuality and relationships.

Throughout this book, we've attempted to define technical words when they first appear in the text. You'll also find a glossary at the back of the book, so you can look up these words and their definitions. In addition, we've gathered an extensive list of resources including books, organizations, support groups, hotlines, and Web sites to help you and your teen deal with specific issues.

Finally, who are we, and why should you trust what we say to you on these pages? We've been happily married to each other since 1967, and we've been sex therapists since 1973. We've team-taught courses on love, relationships, and sex at the college level for more than twenty-five years (during which the social scene of sexuality has changed, to put it mildly). We've led sexuality retreats for ninth-grade teens from both private and public schools for more than a decade. We've worked with parents in workshops around the country, encouraging them and teaching them how to talk with teens about love, relationships, and sex.

But our most important credential (in our opinion) is that we've raised two daughters, now lovely young women in their twenties. We know firsthand what it's like to parent teens in changing, turbulent times. Our journey has been a joyous one. We wish the same for you, and we hope this book will help.

Amy and Charles Miron

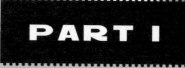

PART I

Steps on the Way to Talking with Your Teen

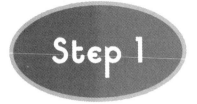

Step 1

DEFINE YOUR VALUES AND GOALS

When our daughters were little, we answered any question they asked as honestly as we could. We tried to respond immediately, keeping the information at a level we felt they could understand. Not just as parents, but as sex educators and therapists, we believed this was the right thing to do and were comfortable with that.

Every once in a while, when a daughter's friend was playing at our house, one of them would ask us a question about sexuality. Our standard response was to refer the friend to her parents and to tell our daughter we'd talk about it later.

One evening, our daughter Lynne asked why we wouldn't answer her questions about sex when she had a friend visiting but would when she was alone. We explained that not all parents agreed about what the right answers were and we wanted to respect whatever values her friends' families had. Therefore, we'd answer her questions—but not her friend's.

When we referred our daughters' friends back to their parents, it saddened us to hear things like, "I can't ask my parents. They won't talk to me about this stuff," or "They keep telling me they'll explain it when I'm older." Maybe those parents wanted to talk with their children but didn't have the information or know-how.

We wrote this book to provide you with accurate information about love, relationships, and sex, and to suggest ways to communicate that information to your teens. But we strongly believe that any and all of this information should be presented within the context of your value system, and with your goals for your teen's sexuality education in mind.

We don't presume to tell you what your values and goals should be. As trained sex therapists and educators, we can help you clarify your values and focus your goals.

Is Sex Good or Bad?

Is sex good or bad? To answer that, let's take a look at another powerful force of nature: fire.

Fire can cook your food. It can heat your home and keep you warm. It can provide light. In a power failure, what's one of the first things you're likely to look for? A book of matches and a candle. We value fire. Without fire, we wouldn't be here; our ancestors couldn't have survived.

Yet if fire gets out of control, our feelings about it change. It becomes a terrifying agent of destruction. It can burn down your house. It can blaze across the landscape, turning everything in its path to cinder. It can kill you.

Is fire good or bad? Neither. Fire just is. If you respect and harness its power, it's a valuable tool. If you abuse it, it can destroy you.

It's the same with sex. Sex isn't good or bad. It just is. When engaged in with respect, sex can be a wonderful, positive experience. It can be great fun—a lifelong source of pleasure and enjoyment. It can nurture a profound bond between two people. It can create new life.

Or sex can ruin your life. The emotional consequences of unhealthy sexual decisions, including low self-esteem, guilt, and depression, can affect your teen's life for years. An unwanted pregnancy can compromise educational, career, or life goals—and maybe even life itself. Some sexually transmitted infections (STIs) can cause great pain. Many are incurable. Some will kill you.

That's why it's important to talk with your teen about love, relationships, and sex—the positive aspects and the negative. Teach him how to harness their power. Teach him how to avoid getting burned. Because, in this case, what your teen doesn't know really can hurt him.

The conversations we suggest you have will take place between at least two people: you and your teen. In later chapters, we'll look at what's going on in the typical teenage mind and body. But let's begin with you, the parent, the person who will probably initiate this dialogue. What are the sexual values that you want to pass on to your teen? What are your goals for her relationships and sexuality education? Before you form your answers, let's consider how culture, society, and religion may have influenced your beliefs.

JUST THE FACTS

Among fifteen- to seventeen-year-olds who have not had sex, 52 percent cite religious or moral beliefs as a "major reason" for their decision to wait.[1]

Cultural and Religious Influences

By "sexuality," we don't just mean the physical act of sexual intercourse. In a broader sense, sexuality includes sexual identity, sexual orientation, sexual behavior, love, affection, relationships, and so much more. Sexuality has an impact on almost every aspect of our lives.

Like eating, sex is a natural, fundamental human activity. In some respects, sexuality education is not so different from those early eating lessons you gave your child. If you take a closer look at what teaching a child to eat really involves, getting the food from plate to mouth is just the beginning.

First, there's the question of what makes an acceptable meal. Most parents aren't pleased to find their child out in the garden eating snails or grasshoppers, yet both are considered delicacies in some parts of the world. Your religious beliefs may put certain foods off limits. In some religions, eating pork is not acceptable. In others, pork is fine but beef is not. Vegetarians may not want their children to eat meat of any kind. Whatever the content, most of us, as concerned parents, are committed to providing a healthy diet for our children.

Then there's the question of utensils. Spoon? Fork? Fingers? Chopsticks? That depends on the type of food that's being eaten, where it's being eaten, and who's eating it.

Table manners don't come naturally, and they vary from family to family. Children need to be coached not to chew with their mouths open or to talk with their mouths full. They need to learn not to put their elbows on the table, not to take food from someone else's plate, or whatever constitutes good manners in your family.

So while eating is a basic human activity, certain aspects of eating are influenced by the social and cultural context in which it's done.

As you plan your child's sexuality education, consider what's important to you, your family, and the world you live in. For example, there's nothing inherently "right" or "wrong" about almost any sexual behavior, with the exception of abusive behaviors. Right and wrong can only be determined within a particular context and set of values.

Your moral and religious beliefs will influence both the way you present sexual information to your children and the type of information you choose to provide. And whether you're conscious of them or not, subtle messages sent by society will influence your decisions.

Your Values

Amusement parks and other attractions usually provide large maps near the entrance so visitors can take a minute to orient themselves. The most important feature is the little red arrow that says, "You are here."

When it comes to your sexual values, where are you? This may seem like a simple question, but many of us have a hard time defining and articulating our sexual values. Maybe we adopted our values from our parents and haven't spent a lot of time thinking about them. Maybe we developed our own values, based on our life experiences, but we haven't really put them into words. Maybe we haven't really needed to—until now, when we're parents who want to have a positive influence on our teens' beliefs, choices, and behaviors.

Try This

Think about your sexual values. Write them down. What do you believe is "right"? What do you believe is "wrong"? Why? Where do your beliefs come from? Are they your personal beliefs, or are they based on what other people have told you or expected of you? Are you satisfied with your sexual values? Are there any you'd like to reconsider or maybe even change?

Perhaps this exercise was easy for you. Perhaps it was very difficult. If you're struggling to clarify your sexual values so you can communicate them to your teen, you may want to talk with your partner, your spiritual leader, your parents, a counselor, or another adult you trust.

You may also find it helpful to consider the list below. It's a set of values often included in sexuality education programs. You don't have to agree with all of them, and you may not agree with any of them. You may think they go too far—or not far enough. No matter how you feel about them, they will start you thinking about language to use and points to make as you talk with your teen about love, relationships, and sex.

VALUES OFTEN INCLUDED IN SEXUALITY EDUCATION PROGRAMS

- Sexuality is a natural and healthy part of living.
- All persons are sexual.
- Sexuality includes physical, ethical, social, spiritual, psychological, and emotional dimensions.

continued ⟶

- Every person has dignity and self-worth.
- Young people should view themselves as unique and worthwhile individuals within the context of their cultural heritage.
- Individuals express their sexuality in varied ways.
- Parents should be the primary sexuality educators of their children.
- Families provide their children's first education about sexuality.
- Families share their values about sexuality with their children.
- In a pluralistic society, people should respect and accept the diversity of values and beliefs about sexuality that exist in a community.
- Sexual relationships should never be coercive or exploitative.
- All children should be loved and cared for.
- All sexual decisions have effects or consequences.
- All persons have the right and the obligation to make responsible sexual choices.
- Individuals, families, and society benefit when children are able to discuss sexuality with their parents and/or other trusted adults.
- Young people develop their values about sexuality as part of becoming adults.
- Young people explore their sexuality as a natural process of achieving sexual maturity.
- Premature involvement in sexual behaviors poses risks.
- Abstaining from sexual intercourse is the most effective method of preventing pregnancy and STD/HIV.
- Young people who are involved in sexual relationships need access to information about health-care services.

From *Guidelines for Comprehensive Sexuality Education, Kindergarten–12th Grade*, 2nd Edition. Copyright © 1996, Sexuality Information and Education Council of the United States (SIECUS), *www.siecus.org*, (212) 819-9770. Used with permission.

Your Goals for Your Teen

You're back in the amusement park, looking at the map and the "You are here" arrow. Where are you when it comes to the sexual values and behaviors you want for your teen?

Try This

Imagine your teen as a fully sexually educated young adult. What qualities would you like to see in him? Write these down. What sexual values would you like him to have? Write these down. What sexual behaviors, if any, are okay? When do they become okay? How would you like your teen to approach dating and relationships now? In three years from now? Five years? Ten? Twenty?

If other adults are sharing the childrearing with you, ask them to create their own lists. Share and compare lists. Keep these lists handy, as they will help guide you.

If you did the "Try This" exercise, you've defined some of your goals for your child's relationships and sexuality education. You've written a description of how you would like your child to behave and what you would like your child to believe at various points in the future. That's an important start. If you didn't do the exercise, you might want to spend some time thinking about the person you'd like your child to become.

Now consider where you are in relation to your goals for your teen. What information and skills have you given her already? What do you still need to teach her? Which model of sexual behavior would you like her to follow: abstinence, delay, or responsible sexual involvement?

- **Abstinence** has traditionally meant not engaging in sexual intercourse until marriage. However, abstinence may mean different things to different people. For example, is someone who engages in oral sex abstinent? As you talk with your teen, you'll need to discuss what abstinence means to each of you and agree on a precise definition.

- **Delayed sexual expression** requires that certain sexual activities be abstained from until conditions other than marriage have been met. This might include reaching a specific age or degree of commitment in a relationship.

- **Responsible sexual involvement** emphasizes *how* a teen will engage in sexual behavior rather than *when*.

Later in the book,* we'll discuss these models in more detail and suggest ways to present them to your child. You probably have an idea of which model you prefer. Hold that thought.

---

* See "Step 5: Choose Your Model and Customize It" (pages 60–75).

The Double Standard

Although it has been pronounced dead many times, the double standard is alive and well. The messages we give our boys about sexuality are often very different from those we give their sisters. Many boys are encouraged to experiment and explore their sexuality, but most girls are given different messages, usually beginning with "Don't."

When a young girl learns that sexual intercourse involves a man putting his penis in her vagina, she may say, "Yuck!" The adult response to this is usually something like, "Oh, sweetie, if you love someone, it can be beautiful." At a tender age, love and sex get tangled together for many little girls.

While this isn't necessarily a bad message, her brother often gets a very different one. Adolescent males may gain status by having sex. In order to succeed in a macho culture, love and sex frequently get separated for males. This can have dire consequences in adolescence (and beyond). A woman may decide to engage in sexual behavior based on the feeling of love. A man may engage in the same sexual acts to gain status.

A young woman is seldom given a right to the same sexual curiosity and experimentation that society grants young men. In most cultures, single men gain status by having sex, while single women lose status by engaging in the same activities.

The double standard has led many people to believe that women are not as sexual as men—or that nice women aren't, anyway. But women have sexual fantasies. Women experience sexual tension. Women masturbate.

Are the messages you plan to give your daughter about sexuality the same ones you plan to give your son?

Try This

Fold a piece of paper in half lengthwise. At the top of one half, write "Daughter." At the top of the other, write "Son." Even if you only have one child, think about your sexuality education goals for both sexes. List your goals in each column. What information do you believe is appropriate for each? How do you want each to handle relationships? What sexual behaviors are okay for each, and at what age? What behaviors are never okay?

Afterward, look at your lists. Are they the same? Why or why not?

Are the sexual standards you expect your daughter to follow the same as those for your son? Talk with your teens about this. Explain your feelings and beliefs. Even if they don't agree with you, they should know where you're coming from.

Your Values vs. Your Partner's Values

Just as we don't make assumptions about what your values should be, we won't pretend to know how your family is constructed. Maybe you've been married to your teen's other parent for many years. Maybe you're a single parent, or you're in a blended family. Maybe you're raising teens with another parent of the same sex. Whatever form your family takes, your teen needs input from all the caring adults in his life, especially when it comes to issues of love, relationships, and sex.

Parents don't always agree on all (or any) of the issues involving the sexuality education of their teen. On those where you disagree, label your differences clearly but respectfully. You might say something like, "Your Mom and I don't agree about such-and-such. I think this way because [give your reason(s)]. You'll need to ask your Mom why she feels the way she does." Even if you don't get along with your teen's other parent(s)—even if you're frustrated, hurt, or angry—it's always in your teen's best interests to talk respectfully about him or her.

Your Values vs. Your Teen's Values

What if your teen's values don't coincide with your own? Can you allow for respectful differences? Are you open to discussing and examining them with your teen? How will you deal with disagreement on various sexual issues? Have a plan of action for handling differences if they do occur.

Your plan might be as simple as inviting your teen to talk and just listening. Or you might agree that each of you gets time to talk without being interrupted by the other. You might each tell where your values come from and why they're important to you.

Later in the book,* we'll offer specific suggestions for handling differences of opinion constructively. For now, just be aware that disagreements probably will happen between you and your teen. They're a normal part of human interaction, and they're almost inevitable when it comes to issues of relationships and sexuality.

Ideally, any conversation on these topics will be productive in some way. It shouldn't be a contest about whose values and goals are "best" or "right." But before you get down to the serious business of talking with your teen about relationships and sexuality,** you'll want to spend some time thinking about your values. Consider the kinds of messages you want to give your teen to help her make decisions that are healthy and right for her.

---

* See "Step 5: Choose Your Model and Customize It" (pages 60–75).

** See "Step 6: Talk with Your Teen" (pages 76–93).

JUST THE FACTS

Fifty-two percent of all teenage girls "strongly agree" that they share the same values with their parents. Forty percent of teen boys feel the same.[2]

Of course, there's no guarantee that your teen will share your beliefs or adhere to the model (abstinence, delay, or responsible involvement) you feel is most appropriate. However, when you express your values clearly and explain why you believe as you do, you increase the chances that your teen will follow your lead.

Love-Sex, Fun-Sex, and Sex-Sex

We've created a simple, nonthreatening vocabulary you can use to start talking about relationships and sexuality with your teen, and also to begin communicating your values.

Despite the fact that ice cream comes in hundreds of exotic flavors—rum raisin, boysenberry ripple, double-chocolate-marshmallow-crunch—there are three standard flavors you can find anywhere in any brand: vanilla, chocolate, and strawberry.

Despite the fact that people have sex for all kinds of reasons and in all kinds of ways, there are three standard "flavors" most of us will experience in an ongoing relationship. We call them "love-sex," "fun-sex," and "sex-sex."

Love-sex is an emotional feeling expressed physically. This kind of sexual encounter is a way of communicating the love two people feel for each other. People often describe this flavor as "making love." Love isn't something that happens overnight. It takes time and commitment. So love-sex can only exist within a loving, respectful relationship that is built over time. It requires both people to be actively in touch with their feelings of love for the other at the time of the sexual encounter. Love-sex will not realize its full expression if either partner is worried about being interrupted, distracted by thinking of other things, pressured for time, or feeling unsafe. It's probably not going to be fully realized if either partner is tired, sick, or worried about STIs or birth control. Love-sex is a deep, meaningful experience. Traditionally, our society values love-sex and places its stamp of approval on this flavor.

Fun-sex can occur within a loving relationship, but it can also be experienced in nonloving relationships. Fun-sex involves the mutual enjoyment of both partners. It's having sex simply because sex can be so much fun. It has a lighter emotional feel to it than love-sex. It may involve a new position or location, or playing with a sex toy or a tickle fight in the middle of having sexual intercourse. It's whatever the partners define as fun on that occasion.

The goal of sex-sex is simply to have an orgasm. You're feeling sexual and you want to climax. It's like scratching an itch. Sex-sex can happen within a loving relationship. Like fun-sex, it does not require love to be experienced. Unlike fun-sex, the goal of sex-sex is essentially the release of sexual tension. People use a myriad of slang expressions that lack tenderness to describe this flavor of sex. The epitome of sex-sex is the quickie, which is often no more than using a partner's body to masturbate.

Although we've described love-sex, fun-sex, and sex-sex as distinct flavors, sometimes they blend together. A couple may start out in a fun-sex experience and get in touch with the deep feeling of love they have for each other, which could change the encounter to love-sex.

Talking with your teen about the three flavors of sex can help you discuss the difference between sex engaged in out of biological urge, curiosity, or experimentation and sex engaged in as emotional expression. For example, you might spend a few minutes watching MTV or a prime-time TV sitcom with your teen. You'll probably see references to sex-sex or fun-sex. Since so much entertainment emphasizes these kinds of sex, your teen might think they're all sex is supposed to be. Take this opportunity to briefly describe the three flavors of sex. If the program you're watching includes jokes about someone having a "hot date," you could ask your teen how he feels about the jokes. You might say, "That sounds to me like sex-sex or fun-sex. What do you think?" Then share your thoughts on the subject.

If a scene in a movie you're watching (or know that your teen has viewed) depicts love-sex, chances are that loving sexual encounter does not include safer sex practices. What a wonderful opportunity to say something like, "That scene seems to show love-sex. Did you ever wonder why they don't show the guy reaching for a condom?" Or, "I believe that in truly loving relationships, partners protect each other from pregnancy and sexually transmitted infections. What do you think?"

UNDERSTAND YOUR TEEN'S PERSONALITY

What happened to that cute baby you used to cuddle, that sweet little girl who came to you with all her innocent secrets? Who is this awkward, moody stranger living in your daughter's room?

At the same time you're asking yourself questions like these, you may also be discovering how exciting the teen years can be. As your daughter gains in strength and understanding and learns new skills, her potential seems to explode in all directions. It's as if she's several people at once. Sometimes you catch glimpses of the playful child you remember, or a hint of the responsible adult she will become. At other times, another personality comes through—one that's resentful, opinionated, even downright obnoxious. The thought of talking to this person about anything—let alone sexuality—is daunting.

It's not just the body that changes as a teen matures sexually. When those hormones kick in, they activate powerful emotions, and a teen's personality starts turning cartwheels. In this chapter, we'll look at what's going on in an adolescent's mind. First, let's consider the world today's teenager lives in to see how the messages and pressures may have changed since you were your child's age. The better you understand your teen and her world, the easier it will be to talk with her.

A Different World

When you were a teen, television, movies, music, and magazines were, by today's standards, pretty mild, although they probably shocked your parents. By contrast, if your teen was watching TV during the 1999/2000 television season, he was exposed to blatant sexual content during 75 percent of prime-time programs and 68 percent of all programming. In only 10 percent of those sexual situations was safer sex represented.[1]

Add the impact of films, music, videos, the Internet, and magazines to that of television, and it becomes evident that children and teens in the United States today learn about sexuality through almost unlimited exposure to sexual scenes containing few or no positive messages about protection and responsibility.[2] If your teen watches the Grammy Awards, he'll see more skin in an hour than you saw at his age in a year.

Just as the TV your teen watches is different from what you watched, his daily life is different as well.

The Miron Model

Over the years, we've created a model of personality development that we find very helpful in understanding how people function. We believe it can help you understand yourself and your teen and communicate more effectively. Our model can also provide a window into the complex motivations that may underlie both your behavior and your teen's.

Look in the mirror. You may think you see one person, but by the time you reach your middle twenties, there are really three of you: the Child, the Adolescent, and the Adult. The Child develops when we're very young, followed at puberty by the Adolescent. As we continue to develop emotionally through our teen years, the Adult should emerge.

Even as we become Adults, the Child and Adolescent aspects of our personalities don't disappear. The thoughts and feelings associated with each of these aspects stay with us and can surface at any time and influence our behavior. They can work well together or be in conflict. For example, consider yourself, right now, reading this book. Your Adult wants to learn more about how to talk with your daughter about love, relationships, and sex. But your Adolescent may be thinking, "I already know all this. Besides, it's time for my favorite TV show," or "I think I'll skip ahead to see if they have any sexy pictures." Meanwhile, your Child may be tapping her fingers, asking, "Are you finished yet? I'm hungry!"

Developmentally, your teen can gain access primarily to the Child or Adolescent parts of her personality. You've probably watched her flip back and forth between these two parts many times. One moment you're talking with a surly Adolescent, and in a flash she's replaced by a giggly Child. One of the greatest challenges in parenting a teen is to help guide her as she develops a healthy, responsible Adult aspect to complement her Child and Adolescent.

When your teen asks a relationship or sexual question that stirs up a variety of feelings in you, our model can help you figure out where those mixed feelings are coming from. Once you know more about the source of your own feelings, you can better understand and respond to your teen.

In the course of parenting, you'll often want to bring your own Child or Adolescent out to play. For example, when your family is at the beach, your Adolescent might join your son in making a bigger sand castle than the family next to you, or your Child might have a water fight with your daughter. But when it comes to sexuality education, you'll want to keep your Adult in charge.

THE MIRON MODEL

THE CHILD: The part of our personality that forms in early childhood. It is the source of wonder and joy, but it can also feel inferior, vulnerable, and powerless. No matter what our chronological age may be, the Child continues to influence many of our thoughts, feelings, and actions.

THE ADOLESCENT: The part of our personality that develops around the time of puberty. Its goals are to become independent, clarify values, explore sexual identity and sexuality, and discover personal strengths and weaknesses. The Adolescent is often creative and full of positive energy, but it can also be insecure, competitive, and rebellious. No matter what our chronological age may be, the Adolescent still influences many of our thoughts, feelings, and actions.

THE ADULT: The part of our personality that emerges as we work through the insecurity, inferiority, and power issues of childhood, as well as the sexual identity and sexuality, independence, and competition issues of adolescence. The Adult has developed an internal definition of self and can appropriately draw upon the positive energy of the Child and Adolescent parts of its personality.

THE CHILD

Picture yourself when you were four or five years old. Try to remember what you were like. That's your Child. No matter how old you are now, that little person is still alive and well inside of you. This aspect of your self is spontaneous, playful, silly, curious—and, at the same time, relies heavily upon others for its welfare.

Childhood is often characterized as one long, happy idyll. All of our needs are met. We have no responsibilities. The most difficult decision we face is what toy to play with next. Mistakes are easily corrected with words like, "Do over." Life is simple and magical.

What's wrong with this picture? Plenty! Even if a child is fortunate enough to be born into a perfectly loving, nurturing environment, childhood is difficult in many ways. Along with that sense of spontaneity and wonder are feelings of bewilderment, powerlessness, frustration, fear, and anxiety.

In childhood, we're little people living in a land of giants. The giants control every aspect of our lives, and we must play by their rules. Even when the rules make no sense to us, we must follow them or be punished.

And there are rules for everything. We must eat what they tell us to eat, not what we like. We can't eat when we're hungry because it may spoil our appetite for dinner. We can't have dessert until we finish our vegetables. We can't turn on the television. We can't cross the street by ourselves. We can't go to school with our older siblings. We have to go to bed before everyone else. We're powerless.

Children approach language literally, with a logic that's more rigid and concrete than a typical adult's. This can cause misunderstandings. If you tell a child that the moon is made of green cheese, he's likely to believe you. Some people in our practice recall being afraid to eat watermelon when they were children. They'd been told that babies came from seeds planted in their mothers' stomachs. They were sure that if they swallowed a watermelon seed, they'd get pregnant. This may seem cute to a doting parent, but to a child trying to make sense of the world, it's confusing and even frightening.

The Child inside of you was shaped by things that happened to you when you were little. While your Child may have accurate recollections of events, it doesn't have the life experience to interpret them accurately. The Child is egocentric—thinking, like all children, that it is the center of the universe. When a parent is grumpy or angry, a child automatically thinks, "I must have done something wrong." The fact that Daddy just lost his job or Mommy got passed over for a promotion doesn't matter. The Child sees itself as the cause of almost everything that happens, good and bad. This is one reason why children blame themselves when their parents divorce.

Your egocentric Child can affect how you feel as a parent. Imagine that your daughter comes home from school, goes into her room, closes the door, and doesn't come out until dinner. At dinner, she gives one-syllable answers to all of your questions, then returns to her room, where she talks to friends on the telephone or uses the computer for the rest of the evening. She grumps when you tell her to go to bed, which she does with hardly a goodnight. Chances are that the Child in you will feel hurt and responsible, wondering what you did to make her mad. The reality may well be that you had little or nothing to do with her mood and behavior.

The Child defines itself based on other people's reactions. If Mommy loves me, I'm lovable. If Daddy doesn't love me, there must be something wrong with me. Since other people have the power to define the Child within us, they also have the power to devastate us. When your teen's girlfriend breaks up with him, it's the Child inside him that feels destroyed and worthless.

You can begin to figure out when your (or your teen's) Child is around by noticing tone of voice, choice of vocabulary, body language and gestures, or the thoughts, feelings, and behaviors that seem to come from the time when you (or your teen) were little. Who do you think ordered that big piece of chocolate cake with chocolate ice cream and chocolate sauce right before dinner? What part of your teen whines and looks at you with such a pitiful face when he really, really, really wants something? Who in you is afraid of those noises you hear at night, even though the dog, who barks at the slightest disturbance, continues to sleep? Who in your teen says "Yuck" at the mention of semen or menstrual blood? Who in both of you has to "go tinkle" or "go to the little boys' room" when you're at a restaurant? Guess who's getting a kick out of writing this right now? You're right—it's our Child.

When you sense that your teen's Child is in charge during a discussion about sexuality, you might table the talk until later, when your teen is back in Adolescent mode.

THE ADOLESCENT

The little person grows bigger, hormones start pumping, the body starts changing, sexual feelings increase, and a new phase of life begins. Your teen's Adolescent begins to develop as your teen's body develops, incorporating new life experiences and perspectives into this aspect of personality.

A primary function of the Adolescent is to discover who she is as an individual. What are her values? Where does she stand in the pecking order among her peers? What is her sexual orientation? How should she handle this new and changing body? What are her limits? Are there limits?

The Adolescent is struggling to break out of the cocoon of childhood. Children define themselves in relation to others in the family: "Daddy's little girl," "Yoshi's big brother." In order to develop as an individual, the Adolescent has to break out of that cocoon. Psychologically, adolescents start to separate from their families. While parents still play an essential role in their lives, peers become increasingly important. As teens grow out from under the shadow of their families of origin, their parents lose control over many of their actions.

When you understand that your teen is seeking more independence, you can begin to give her more choices about things you feel are appropriate. Reinforce what you believe to be positive, healthy decisions. Seek her opinion whenever possible. While your teen's need for independence is great, so is her need for your approval. It may not seem that way at times, but please don't forget that it is.

The Adolescent, in you as well as in your teen, hasn't established an independent sense of self. It depends on the constant comparison of itself to others. It discovers its strengths and weaknesses through social competition. It competes with peers to find out who's strongest, who's smartest, who has the best body or coolest clothes, who can drink the most beer . . . the list goes on and on. The stage on which this drama unfolds simply changes as we grow older. It's the Adolescent in you that worries about who has the biggest house on the block, whose kid is the brightest or is the best athlete, or who has the highest score in the bowling league. In the world of the Adolescent, there's constant comparison, measuring, and testing.

In teens' lives, these Adolescent competitions often take a sexual turn, like comparing to see whose penis or breasts are bigger, who gets pubic hair soonest, and who can get the most dates or go farthest sexually. Like wrestling to see who's strongest, or running to see who's fastest, this sexual exploration has the goal of establishing one's place or status among peers.

Because both you and your teen have competing Adolescent aspects, be aware of the circumstances under which you let your own Adolescent emerge. It might be okay to let your Adolescent out to play with your teen's Adolescent in one-on-one basketball. It might be okay to take your Adolescent shopping with your teen (as long as your Adult is in charge of the credit card). But try not to relive your teen years through your son or daughter. We've known parents who have tried to impose their insecure Adolescent onto their teens' Adolescent. A mother who was shy as a teen wanted her daughter to be popular. A father who gained status when he was a teen through dating and sexual activity couldn't understand why his son wasn't ready to date. Stand back and let your teen's Adolescent develop in a way that's right for her.

Adolescent competition can cause problems in the relationship between you and your teen. Your Adolescent may need to feel more powerful than someone else. If that person is your teen, your Adolescent may try to put her down or diminish her accomplishments.

Adolescent Development At-a-Glance

Our model has helped many parents and teens to better understand themselves and each other. This chart is provided for times when you want a quick overview of what's happening in your teen's life at a particular stage.

Each teen is an individual with a unique personality and special interests, likes, and dislikes. In general, however, there is a series of developmental tasks that everyone faces during the adolescent years.

A teenager's development can be divided into three stages: early, middle, and late adolescence. This chart describes the normal feelings and behaviors for each stage. Teenagers will naturally vary slightly from these descriptions. If a teenager seems very different, it may be appropriate to consult with a mental health professional.

continued ⟶

Based on material developed by the American Academy of Child & Adolescent Psychiatry (AACAP). Used with permission.

Early Adolescence (12–14 years)

Movement Toward Independence

- struggle with sense of identity
- moodiness
- improved abilities to use speech to express oneself
- more likely to express feelings by action than by words
- close friendships gain importance
- less attention shown to parents, with occasional rudeness
- realization that parents are not perfect; identification of their faults
- search for new people to love in addition to parents
- tendency to return to childish behavior, fought off by excessive activity
- peer group influence interests and clothing styles

Sexuality

- girls ahead of boys
- same-sex friends and group activities
- shyness, blushing, and modesty
- show-off qualities
- greater interest in privacy
- experimentation with body (masturbation)
- worries about being normal

Ethics and Self-Direction

- rule- and limit-testing
- occasional experimentation with cigarettes, marijuana, and alcohol
- capacity for abstract thought

Middle Adolescence (14–17 years)

Movement Toward Independence

- self-involvement, alternating between unrealistically high expectations and poor self-concept
- complaints that parents interfere with independence

continued ➝

Based on material developed by the American Academy of Child & Adolescent Psychiatry (AACAP). Used with permission.

- extremely concerned with appearance and with one's own body
- feelings of strangeness about one's self and body
- lowered opinion of parents, withdrawal of emotions from them
- effort to make new friends
- strong emphasis on the new peer group, with the group identity of selectivity, superiority, and competitiveness
- periods of sadness as the psychological loss of the parents takes place
- examination of inner experiences, which may include writing a diary

Sexuality
- concerns about sexual attractiveness
- frequently changing relationships
- movement toward heterosexuality with fears of homosexuality
- tenderness and fears shown toward opposite sex
- feelings of love and passion

Ethics and Self-Direction
- development of ideals and selection of role models
- more consistent evidence of conscience
- greater capacity for setting goals
- interest in moral reasoning

Late Adolescence (17–19 years)

Movement Toward Independence
- firmer identity
- ability to delay gratification
- ability to think ideas through
- ability to express ideas in words
- more developed sense of humor
- stable interests
- greater emotional stability
- ability to make independent decisions

continued →

Based on material developed by the American Academy of Child & Adolescent Psychiatry (AACAP). Used with permission.

- ability to compromise
- pride in one's work
- self-reliance
- greater concern for others

Sexuality
- concerned with serious relationships
- clear sexual identity
- capacities for tender and sensual love

Ethics and Self-Direction
- capable of useful insight
- stress on personal dignity and self-esteem
- ability to set goals and follow through
- acceptance of social institutions and cultural traditions
- self-regulation of self-esteem

Based on material developed by the American Academy of Child & Adolescent Psychiatry (AACAP). Used with permission.

THE ADULT—AND THE GROWN-UP

The rapid and sometimes uncomfortable physical growth of the teen years is preparing your son or daughter for sexual maturity. But sexual maturity doesn't automatically signal psychological and emotional maturity. Physical development without corresponding psychological development leads to that curious creature we call the Grown-up—an adult body powered by an Adolescent's or Child's personality and emotional limitations. There are important differences between an Adult and a Grown-up.

- An Adult has largely resolved the inferiority and powerlessness issues of childhood. Adults consider themselves the equals of other people—neither better nor worse. A Grown-up, however, must constantly compete to prove how powerful he is (as the Adolescent), or seek protection, attention, and support from others (as the Child).

- An Adult has resolved most of the independence, sexual identity, and competition issues of adolescence. Adolescents, and by extension Grown-ups, need the mirror of other people to define who and what they are. A Grown-up believes, "I need to have lots of friends and be popular to prove I'm likable." An Adult no longer requires the reflection of others to have a positive sense of self; it now comes from within.

- An Adult can decide on the best action to take without reference to others. A Grown-up's actions, however, are frequently motivated by the Adolescent's need to conform or to rebel.

To illustrate how these different parts of our personality relate to sexual attitudes and behaviors, let's consider the subject of masturbation. Someone whose Child is in charge may think, "I must be bad because Daddy gets mad when I touch my penis." The person whose Adolescent is in charge may think, "I know I shouldn't do this, but I'm going to anyway, because everyone else does it." A Grown-up may adopt either of these conflicted attitudes about masturbation. But someone whose Adult is in charge is likely to think of masturbation as an activity that he can engage in (or not), depending on his beliefs or inclination, or its impact on his partner.

Becoming a Grown-up is easy. All it takes is time and imitation. That's why teens need help making a successful transition to becoming responsible Adults. They need guidance to resolve crucial issues like sexual values and what forms of sexual expression are acceptable. They need support as they deal with strong new emotions and learn to make appropriate, positive, healthy choices, sexual and otherwise. These are some of the most important functions of parenting. How can we gradually take the training wheels off the bicycle to foster independent travel? How do we get a teen's attention and respect? When and how are these all-important conversations about love, relationships, and sex going to take place?

Using the Model

In "Step 6: Talk with Your Teen," we'll help you find answers to these questions. We'll suggest ways of sidestepping potential conflicts and relating to your teen without patronizing him. We'll show you how to bring up relationship and sexuality issues in ways that are natural, nonthreatening, and even fun. But before you sit down to talk with your teen, let's learn a little more about some potential trouble spots in dealing with the Child and the Adolescent in both of you.

POWER STRUGGLES

Most teens learn about their new powers by pushing against authority. For the parent who suddenly finds her every statement challenged and every suggestion met with suspicion, this can be very trying. It becomes easier (although never easy) when you can understand the goal of your teen's Adolescent.

Most parents probably measure their success (and power) by the outcome of their efforts. When you go to your boss and ask to be paid overtime for the extra hours she asked you to put in during the weekend, you aren't going to be placated by a nice speech about how important your work is to the company. If you don't get the money, the Adolescent part of you will probably feel like you've lost. When your neighbor finally agrees not to let his barking dog out until 9:00 A.M., your Adolescent will probably feel powerful—you've won.

The Adolescent in your teen, on the other hand, doesn't necessarily expect to win—at least, not in the same way an adult does. For example, let's say that a father insists that his sixteen-year-old daughter be home by midnight. This results in a long, heated argument. "Nobody else has a curfew!" she complains . . . but she comes home at 11:58 P.M.

The father will probably interpret this as a win. But does the teen feel that she has lost? A part of her probably won't. Simply engaging in the long confrontation may have made the Adolescent in her feel powerful. The Adolescent measures power not only by the outcome, but also by the process.

Beneath that rebellious attitude you sometimes find in your teen, there's still her Child, who fears she lacks the capacity to control her own life. That sense of powerlessness is still very active, especially in younger teens. The teen arguing about curfew probably knew all along that she'd end up having to give in, but her Adolescent forced an authority figure to invest a big chunk of time and energy in battling with her. In her terms, this is a sign that she's becoming more powerful.

If you find that you're spending big chunks of time arguing with your teen, the Adolescent in you may be cooperating with the Adolescent in your teen to keep a power struggle going. Perhaps your own Adolescent has sensed the growing strength of your teen's Adolescent and feels threatened. Whatever the reason, when the Adolescent in you gets hooked by your teen's Adolescent, no matter what the topic of the fight or the merits of your teen's position, your Adolescent can't or won't give in. That's a lose-lose position for both of you.

As you gain more understanding of your own Adolescent as well as your teen's, you'll be able to figure out better ways for your Adult to help your teen. Instead of battling over issues, you can encourage the growing power of your teen's Adolescent in constructive ways. For example, if your teen asks for a hike in her baby-sitting or lawn-mowing pay, or constructively stands up to a teacher about a grade, you can note her accomplishment and support her assertiveness.

THE NEED FOR ATTENTION

Confrontations with authority figures are often gambits for attention. When a child seeks attention, he'll simply ask for it: "Look at me, Mommy! See what I can do!" When he becomes a teen, such naked expression of need is not acceptable to his Adolescent, but the need for your attention may be just as strong. He'll get it however he can—by seeking positive recognition, or by engaging in negative power struggles. Either way, your focus is on him, and that's what he wants.

The more positive attention he gets, the less negative attention he'll need. Build in positive time with your teen. Watch a movie he's interested in. Listen to music with him. Go for a walk. Play a game. Seek his opinions. Ask what he thinks about the dog's latest behavior problem or a current news event—anything. Take an exercise or art class together. Ask him to teach you something on the computer. If you put your Adult's mind to it, you can think of many ways to show positive attention, no matter how busy and demanding your schedule is.

Teens also crave attention from other teens. In some Latin countries, young people traditionally gather in the town square in the evening for the *paseo,* a leisurely stroll during which they check each other out. The same kind of ritual goes on in our culture in shopping malls every day of the week. Groups of teenagers roam the concourses, keeping a sharp eye out for other teens. A group of girls passing a group of boys may seem to be carefully indifferent, but everything about them, from hair and clothing to posture, advertises their Adolescents crying out to be noticed.

SELF-CENTEREDNESS

Children are often so uninterested in their appearance that it's hard to get them to comb their hair, tuck in their shirts, or wash their hands. In adolescence, appearance may become all-important. Many teens are constantly preening and posturing—trying out dramatic new hairstyles, clothing, and attitudes. It's as if they're always on stage, playing to an audience of their peers.

From your teen's Adolescent perspective, that's exactly what's going on. Suffering from agonies of self-consciousness, the insecure Child and egocentric Adolescent in your teen assume that everyone else is just as aware of his perceived shortcomings as he is. Your son may refuse to go to the school dance because everyone will see how clumsy he is. Your daughter may insist she can't go to class with that huge pimple on her cheek.

Complaints from other family members about having to listen to a certain rock group being played over and over are likely to be met with the Adolescent's disbelief. How can anyone not see that this is the best music ever written? Other siblings may grumble about his hogging the bathroom, telephone, or computer. The Adolescent is often so absorbed in what he is doing that he may not recognize the impact of his behavior on other people.

As a parent, you can teach both the Child and the Adolescent in your teen that he isn't the center of the universe or the family—just an important part. Family life is where the Child and the Adolescent learn to cooperate and become responsible members of a community.

For example, if your teen is playing music at a volume you think is too loud, your Adolescent might say, "I can't hear myself think. Turn down that awful music!" Your teen's Adolescent, who doesn't like being told what to do, might respond, "But I love this group [so everyone should love them]. They've got to be played loud." Your Adolescent, upset that your teen isn't obeying you, might insist, "I SAID turn the music DOWN!" The power struggle has begun.

Instead, let your Adult handle the situation. Your goal as a parent in this situation may be twofold: First, you want your teen to lower the volume. Second, you'd like your teen to learn to be considerate. Knowing your teen likes this group, your Adult might say, "I know you love that group played loudly, but it's interfering with what I'm trying to do." Your teen may still respond with, "I have a right to enjoy my music, and this band is supposed to be played loud." To which the Adult in you could say, "We need to figure out a solution that works for both of us. How about if we get you some headphones?"

FEELING INVINCIBLE

As your teen's Adolescent begins to experiment with its new abilities, the childhood sense of powerlessness may give way to a reckless sense of invulnerability. Not only can your daughter drive; at times, she really believes she can push the speedometer past 90 and still stop on a dime. And your son knows he can ride his skateboard down the middle of the street—he'll never get hit by a car.

At these moments, when a teen is breathing the heady air of new achievement, anything seems possible. The denial mechanism is very strong. "Other people may lose control of their cars and go over the guardrail, but not me," says the seductive voice of new power. "I know what I'm doing. I'm in complete control."

This it-can't-happen-to-me attitude can be very dangerous—especially when it affects sexual decisions. "People like me don't get sexually transmitted infections," the voice says. Or "Other teens get pregnant, but I know I won't." The best defense against that seductive voice is to give your teen the facts about sexual risk and responsibility.

GOING TO EXTREMES

The emerging Adolescent in your teen can be incredibly reasonable, resourceful, logical, and mature much of the time. You'll marvel as you watch her budding Adult handle challenging situations with grace. Then, all at once and seemingly out of nowhere, your rational teen becomes insensitive, self-absorbed, and highly emotional.

The seesaw of teen emotions finds highly dramatic forms of expression. The Child in your teen seeks attention. The Adolescent takes attention-seeking to the next level: melodrama. When the Adolescent is in charge, nothing is simply bad. It's awful, terrible, horrid, disastrous. Infatuations and crushes are short-lived but intense. Your daughter isn't just in love with the new kid at school; she's madly in love. A friend is no longer just a friend but a best friend. And if that best friend has lunch with someone else, your daughter hates her. There's often little middle ground. And that's where you as a parent come in: guiding your teen toward understanding her emotions, letting her know that even if she feels something very, very strongly, that doesn't necessarily make it so.

A dangerously thin anorexic believes she's fat. A gifted child haunted by perfectionism feels stupid. Feelings aren't always based in reality. And even when they are, it helps to step back and let our rational thoughts inform our feelings. That's not an easy lesson for any brain to learn, let alone one bathed in hormones. But it's an important lesson for Adolescents of all ages.

So what do you do when your daughter insists that it's the end of the world because she's on the B squad of the soccer team? Or your son is convinced that his social life is over because the most popular girl in school put him down? Here's a suggestion: Ask your teen to imagine a scale of badness from 1 to 100. One hundred is as bad as life could ever be—for example, lying in a hospital bed on life support without any hope of recovery, aware of everything around you yet unable to communicate. Ask your teen to define her own 100. Then have her use it as a yardstick to measure any bad thing life throws her way. Being ignored is bad, but on a scale of 1 to 100, how bad? Sure, it's on the badness scale, and it deserves a number, but how high a number?

INDEPENDENCE VS. THE NEED TO BELONG

Your teen's search for identity pulls his Adolescent in two different directions. There's the desire to be unique, to express his individuality—sometimes in the most dramatic way possible. At the same time, the Adolescent in your teen feels a strong need to belong.

Many psychologists and sociologists believe that the cliques formed by teens are a substitute for the family. Gaining independence from the family is the goal of the Adolescent, so teens may look to peers for support, approval, and a sense of belonging. Within cliques, there are rigid standards of conformity. To be different can be devastating. If everyone is wearing a certain style, your teen's Adolescent just has to have it, too.

Consider, for example, body piercing and tattooing. While some people enjoy them as art forms and use them to make a personal statement, piercings and tattoos can also be a means of rebelling against mainstream values, getting attention, and establishing membership in a clique—a statement of both conformity and individuality. Within teen cliques, there's a certain amount of competitiveness and jockeying for position. A teen with one body piercing or tattoo is outdone by another with several, or a single bigger one. Mine is bigger than yours.

Talk with your teen. Listen to what he says. You might explain that you understand the desire to belong to a group—you feel it, too. But there has to be a balance. When do you listen to the voice of the group, and when do you heed your own inner voice?

Try This

Ask your teen to "just suppose" that friends have asked her to do the following things. Then ask if she would go along. If you want honest answers, be an Adult—listening respectfully, calmly sharing your values. If your teen says, "Sure, I'd cut school/go for a joy ride," don't let your Child or Adolescent respond, "How could you!?" or "I can't believe you'd be that dumb!" Ask your teen to tell you why she feels that way. Then state your own position and briefly explain it.

Just suppose a friend asked you to . . .

- cut school
- make crank phone calls
- smoke cigarettes
- find pornography on the Internet
- try marijuana
- steal a car and go for a joy ride
- have a dragon tattooed on your leg
- drink beer at a party
- participate in casual sex games at a party

The list can go on and on, and you can use these examples or others of your choosing. You can add any issue you want your teen to think about. Each can serve as a conversation starter about individual vs. group values.

UNDERSTAND YOUR TEEN'S SEXUAL DEVELOPMENT

This step explores children's sexual development from infancy through puberty and looks more closely at the related social and emotional changes your teen is going through. Each of these stages is complex, and we don't attempt to treat them in depth here.* Our goal is to show that your teen's sexual identity and awareness have existed in a continuum of changing thoughts, feelings, and behaviors, starting from when he was in the womb until now.

Infancy

Humans are sexual even before birth. Many pregnant women (and their partners) have been surprised by an ultrasound showing a baby boy's erect penis. If there were ways to measure it, we'd likely find that a baby girl's clitoris is similarly stimulated. Once born, boys commonly have their first erections seconds after delivery. The vaginas of newborn girls will lubricate. These responses continue to occur several times a day while the infant is sleeping. Infant boys may develop erections when their diaper is removed or when they need to urinate. Girls probably lubricate vaginally just as frequently.

Psychologist Erik Erikson noted that basic learning about relationships starts taking place during infancy. Will the infant learn to trust that her needs will be met, or will she learn to mistrust the world? These life lessons are taught when the infant is loved, touched, cuddled, and held—or ignored and abused. Will someone change her diaper when it's dirty? Feed her when she's hungry? Comfort her when she cries? Depending on how they respond to these basic needs, parents teach the infant to trust or mistrust others.

---

* More detailed information is found in "Issue 1: Female Sexual Development" (pages 119–134) and "Issue 2: Male Sexual Development" (pages 135–143).

Lessons about sexuality also begin in infancy. When you take off a baby's diaper, both boys and girls frequently reach straight for their genitals. Why? Because it feels good. It's an infantile form of masturbation. Was it okay for your daughter to explore her vulva? For your son to touch his penis? Children should be taught the correct names for body parts. These lessons provided the foundation of your teen's early sexuality education.

Early Childhood

From ages two to five, most boys and girls continue to engage in variations on the exploratory self-stimulation of infancy, although this is not yet the masturbation to orgasm of later years. Masturbation is common well before puberty.

Some parents who find small children masturbating may say things like, "If you play with your penis too much, it's going to fall off." Statements like these are designed to control children's behavior by frightening them. As you start talking with your teen about sexual behavior, you have the opportunity to correct earlier false or misleading messages you may have sent. For example, you might say something like, "When you were little, I told you that if you played with your penis too much it would fall off. I'm sure you know by now that isn't true, and I wish I hadn't told you it was. I promise to tell you the truth from now on."

By age three or four, children have very strong ideas of what a boy or girl is or isn't supposed to do. In our family, we often chuckle about how we thought we were raising our daughters in a gender-neutral home. Charles would cook dinner or do laundry, and Amy would teach at the college or counsel in the office. We told our daughters specifically that they could grow up to be anything. We were smug in our feelings that we had done our job. Our daughters knew the difference between a Phillips head screwdriver and a slotted one. They loved playing with trucks and could throw a ball with the best of the neighborhood boys. One day, while we were waiting for a blood test at a local hospital, a nurse came to talk to our daughters. She asked our five-year-old, Jill, if she wanted to be a doctor when she grew up. To our shock, Jill responded, "Oh, I can't be a doctor. Boys are doctors. Girls are nurses." So much for our gender-neutral environment!

It's true that children learn mostly from their families, but the world at large is a master teacher as well. All the doctors our daughters knew were men, and the nurses were women. The same was true in the books they read and the TV shows and movies they watched. The message they were getting was consistent, even if their mom and dad said something different.

SEXUAL EXPLORATION GAMES

Young children are naturally curious about their own bodies as well as other children's. They often play "doctor" or "house" as an excuse to explore each other's genitals.

Sex play between children is normal. It happens between kids of the other sex, and it happens between kids of the same sex. Childhood friends are often the same sex. This kind of sex play doesn't "make" a child straight or gay. It has not been shown to influence sexual orientation in later life.

As sex therapists, we've found that the way people remember their childhood sexual exploration games often depends on whether they were discovered by an adult—and what the adult's reaction was. Some recall a parent screaming, "WHAT do you think you're DOING?" Others were spanked, deprived of privileges, or punished in other ways. In our practice, we've seen adults who are still dealing with the guilt of being, quite literally, caught with their pants down.

It isn't uncommon for siblings and other young family members to engage in sexual exploration games. This can lead to guilt later, when people recall their explorations in light of deep-seated incest taboos. But small children haven't learned these taboos, and body exploration with a sibling isn't a problem for a child—it's a simple matter of kids in the same family being accessible to each other.

It's natural for children to sexually explore with others who are close to them in age—within a couple of years. But sex play among children who are more than a couple of years apart may signal a problem. It's the play part of sex play that children are interested in. Older children may be more interested in the sex part. Children engaging in sex play generally don't insert anything into each other's bodies. When a child tells a parent about someone attempting to insert an object or a finger into an anus or a vagina—or a penis into any body opening—parents need to talk to the child calmly, find out exactly what happened, and consult their pediatrician immediately for further guidance.

Your teen may have engaged in sex play when she was younger. You might find a teachable moment, such as seeing two young children playing together, and casually ask if your teen played "doctor" when she was little. Add something like, "You know, most kids do." Both boys and girls need to be reassured that this was probably normal and harmless.

Perhaps, at some point in the past, you interrupted a childhood sexual exploration game, and your reaction wasn't what you now wish it had been. It's not too late to clear that up. Let your teen know that what she was doing back then was a product of natural, healthy curiosity, despite what you might have said in the heat of the moment.

NUDITY

At some point in early childhood, most parents will want to address the topic of nudity. What you tell your child will depend on your own values and comfort levels.

Some parents would never allow a young child to see them undressed or allow the child to go nude in mixed company. For these families, it's out of the bath and into clothes immediately. Other families are comfortable with partial nudity in the privacy of their home. Dads and boys can be seen in their boxers, and moms and girls in their bras and panties.

Children learn about their bodies and whether nudity is okay through how the family handles a host of daily activities. Showering, bathing, changing clothes, using the toilet, and getting ready for bed are all stages on which the question of nudity, as well as many other issues, unfold. Think about how you handled these issues with your child. Have you been sending the messages you'd like to send?

Middle Childhood

In the early school years, approximately from ages six to nine, many children continue to masturbate and explore each other's bodies. Whether or not you think it's okay to masturbate in private, or to engage in sex play, let your children know your values. Try not to attach shame or blame to these behaviors.

The age differences involved and what the children are doing will determine whether their sex play is normal curiosity, inappropriate, or abusive. Typically, exploration is done with someone in the same age group. If you have any questions concerning sex play you've found out about, seek professional guidance. Talk with your pediatrician, religious leader, school counselor, or another professional you trust.

Children in middle childhood will probably start asking where babies come from. Sometimes that's all they really want to know—*where* babies come from, not *how* they are made. If that's the case, it's usually enough to give a brief response. For example, you might say, "Babies come from inside their mothers." If a child asks, "Where inside?" you could say, "They grow in a part of the mother's body called the uterus." If he asks, "How do they get out?" you could say, "They come out an opening in the mother's body called the vagina." Always use the correct names for body parts. Babies don't grow in a stomach; they grow in a uterus.

Many parents panic when they hear the "where-do-babies-come-from" question. They respond with more information than the child wants or needs. Listen to what your child is asking. Find out what he already knows. You might say, "That's a great question. What made you ask?" Then give brief, simple, honest, age-appropriate answers to his specific questions, without elaborating or overexplaining.

What if he asks how babies are made? A reasonable answer for this age group might be: "Men make sperm in their testicles. Women have eggs in their ovaries. Sometimes a man and a woman decide to enjoy each other's bodies. One way for grown-ups to do this is for the woman to receive a man's penis in her vagina. After a while, sperm comes out of the man's penis and travels up her vagina into her uterus. If one of her eggs is ready, a sperm and an egg get together, and from that a baby will grow."

What if he reacts with disgust? You might reassure him by saying, "Lots of kids your age feel that way. That's okay. When you're an adult, you may change your mind."

Build your values into your response. Whatever you say, be honest. For example, if you think that only married adults *should* have babies, that's what you should tell your child. But if you say that only married adults *can* have babies, your child is bound to encounter a teen mother or an unmarried couple with a baby sooner or later. He'll be confused, and he may be less trusting of what you tell him after that. Consider saying something like: "You might decide to have a baby someday. I believe that only adults who are married to each other should have babies. Some people don't feel this way, but I do, and here's why . . . ." Your explanation can reflect your values.

Puberty

One minute your child is playing with her toys, and the next she's fighting for the right to go out on dates. What's happening? Hormones. Puberty is when hormones start to hum. As they pump through your child's body, it begins to take on the physical characteristics of an adult, including the ability to reproduce.

Girls usually enter puberty two to two-and-a-half years earlier than boys—around ages eight to thirteen. Once puberty starts for boys, they continue to grow and develop long after girls stop, which is why most adult men are taller than most adult women.

With all the rapid body changes going on, many teens wonder whether they are normal. If your teen (or preteen) is feeling self-conscious, offer reassurance. Explain that her body is simply preparing her to be an adult. You might say something like, "I know that puberty feels really strange sometimes. But I promise you'll get used to the changes in your body, even if it doesn't seem that way right now."

An early hint of puberty is when your child starts outgrowing clothes faster than you can blink. Fat cells are redistributed in your daughter's body—first behind her nipples to cause the budding of her breasts, and then on her hips, thighs, and buttocks. Hair appears under her arms and in her pubic area. Your son's testicles and penis grow, along with underarm and pubic hair. Facial hair sprouts as peach fuzz, first on his upper lip, then on the rest of his face and body. His voice deepens and—unlike girls, who usually spread out in the hips—he develops broader shoulders, longer legs, and narrower hips.

These changes aren't orchestrated in a symphony of smoothness and grace, and they happen for each teen at different times and to different degrees. But generally the arms, legs, hands, and feet grow first, causing your teen to look gangly and awkward.

One day, when you go to give your teen a hug, you notice that she isn't that sweet-smelling baby you used to snuggle. Hormones cause the sweat glands to enlarge and become more active, especially under the arms and in the genital area. Scientists believe that these smells once served as sexual attractants, and at some level they may still play a similar role. Teens, who are already likely to be self-conscious about these new smells, are barraged with ads telling them that their armpits and genitals should smell like a garden. This is nonsense, but even so, adolescents should bathe regularly and start using underarm deodorant or antiperspirant.

Many adolescents break out in pimples during puberty. Your teen may get whiteheads, blackheads, pimples, and painful bumps not only on his face, but also on his neck, shoulders, back, and chest as well. How can you help? First, suggest that he not wash his face too much. Acne isn't caused by dirt, so cleaning his face twice a day with a mild soap or a product made specifically for pimples is sufficient. Tell him that washing his face much more than that can aggravate the condition. Urge him to leave his pimples alone—squeezing them can lead to infections and scarring. If he's really distressed by his acne, or if he has a serious case that won't heal, consider taking him to a dermatologist.

JUST THE FACTS

About 85 percent of the people in the U.S. between ages twelve and twenty-five suffer with various degrees of acne.[1]

Teens often worry about the timing of their sexual development. Girls experience their first period, or menarche, at different ages. Similarly, boys experience their first ejaculation with semen at various ages, either while they're masturbating or during sleep in a wet dream. Being at either end of the development spectrum can be worrisome for a teen. If your daughter develops breasts earlier than her friends, she may be teased by her peers and encouraged by older children to start experimenting sexually. If she's slower to develop than her friends, she may be made fun of as well. Boys who develop early fare a bit better than their sisters. They are often given roles of leadership by peers as well as adults. A common problem for kids of either sex who develop early is that adults often expect more of them than of their slower-developing friends.

Perhaps the two most important messages you can give your teen during puberty are: 1) Puberty starts and ends at different ages for different people, and 2) Everyone's body changes at its own pace. There's no "right" or "wrong" way to go through puberty.

Many teens experiment with masturbation, this time with orgasm as a goal. Sexual fantasies are common. If you're uncomfortable talking with your teen about masturbation, you're not alone. Of all the subjects associated with sexual behavior, masturbation is the one adults are least comfortable with. At a minimum, try to communicate that masturbation is normal. It's universal. It won't make you walk funny, and nobody can tell by looking at you how often you've indulged. If your values permit, let your teen know that masturbation done in private is a safe way to release sexual tension and learn how one's body responds.* In any conversation with your teen about this topic, let your Adult take the lead.**

FRIENDS AND FIRST RELATIONSHIPS

Puberty also marks a turning point in your teen's social development. It's hard to know ahead of time how your teen will develop socially, but it helps to understand that some fairly predictable behavior patterns emerge at about the same time as hormonal and sexual changes occur.

It's not uncommon for a teen's early social life to develop around a clique, or a special group of friends, usually of the same sex. Peer pressure is at an all-time high. Suddenly, your teen, who once shared everything with you, seems only interested in being with his friends. His door stays closed (and so may his ears) except to them. You may feel disheartened and hurt, but try not to worry too much. He's doing what he's supposed to be doing at this stage of life. Breaking away from his family of origin and establishing closer relationships with peers is part of what being a teen is all about.

Sometimes it's easier to separate from someone you love when you're angry—which may account for the sarcasm and hostility that often color teens' interactions with their parents. If you don't like the way your teen is handling this period of separation, talk with him about it. You might say something like, "I understand how important your friends are. But it hurts me when you shut me out and talk to me with that angry tone of voice. Is there anything you're angry at me about? If there is, tell me and I'll work on it. Meanwhile, I'd appreciate your talking with me without so much anger."

It's likely that the cliques in your child's school are tight. By the sixth grade, and possibly sooner, your son or daughter can probably tell you who's in which group. As teens go through middle school, cliques join together and start to form crowds. Suddenly, the other sex is more available, and group dating becomes common. A bunch of teens may go the movies or the mall or just hang out together. Some may pair up, but for the most part they stay in a group.

"Going together" at this age usually means holding hands, passing notes, calling, and/or sending emails. Sometimes it's simply a matter of one person liking another. If there's a school dance, adolescents who are "going

---

* If you'd like to tell your teen that masturbation is okay but you just can't get the words out, see the "Try This" exercise on page 159.

** See "The Miron Model" on pages 19–27.

together" may dance together some. Some kids will tell their parents that they're "going with" so-and-so; others won't. If you want to keep the lines of communication open, talk with your teen without teasing her. Teasing is almost guaranteed to cut off the information flow.

If your teen hasn't yet mentioned that she's going with anyone, you could ask something like, "Are any of your friends going together?" If she says no, you could follow up with, "I hope you'll talk with me when you start wanting to go with someone. It's an exciting time, and I'd love to share it with you."

In time, hanging out and going together lead to dating. And with dating, the potential for sexual involvement becomes greater. Make a real effort to nurture your relationship with your teen before she starts dating. Find out what's going on in her life. Get to know her friends. Have a lot of "little" talks about dating, relationships, peer pressure, and other topics that arise naturally. Keep the lines of communication open, and share your values whenever it seems appropriate. You're laying the groundwork now for more serious conversations later.

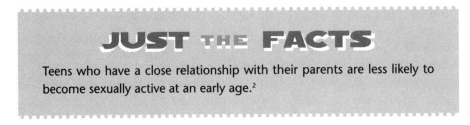

JUST THE FACTS

Teens who have a close relationship with their parents are less likely to become sexually active at an early age.[2]

UNDERSTAND YOUR TEEN'S RELATIONSHIPS

Although many things have changed since you were a teen, some things haven't. Just as you did when you entered middle or high school, your teen has probably begun to experience his first romantic relationships. How he handles these relationships and what he learns from them will depend on the interplay of his feelings, perspectives, personality, and values with those of his partners and friends—and with your own.

What Is Intimacy?

Intimacy, like love, means different things to different people. What does it mean to you? What are the qualities you think make a relationship intimate, as opposed to casual? These are the qualities people have mentioned most often to us over the years:

- trusting and feeling trusted
- mutual respect
- honesty
- loyalty
- concern for each other
- sharing thoughts and feelings
- shared interests
- unconditional, nonjudgmental acceptance
- sharing affection

What about sex? Are you surprised that sex isn't on our list? Some people assume that sexual behavior is a necessary component of an intimate relationship. It's an easy assumption to make. Advertisers refer to lingerie as "intimate apparel." People who are trying to be delicate about finding out whether a couple is sexually involved may ask, "Are they intimate?"

But intimacy and sexual expression are two different things. You can be sexual without being intimate. Strangers can trigger intense sexual attraction.

And you can also be intimate without being sexual. People can have very close relationships without any sexual feelings.

Refraining from sexual expression doesn't detract from intimacy, and adding sexual activity to a relationship doesn't necessarily make it more intimate. Intimacy is a state of mind, not a physical act. This is important for teens to know as sexual feelings begin to play a role in their relationships. You might ask your teen to make a list of the qualities she associates with intimacy. Use this as an opportunity to open a discussion of intimacy and sexual expression.

Your Teen's Peer Group

Think of your teen's various relationships as a group of four concentric circles—circles of different sizes that share the same center. In this case, the center is your teen.

The farther a circle is from the center, the less intimate the relationship. The outside circle represents acquaintances—people your teen might pass in the hall at school and occasionally say hello to but doesn't really know. Because this is the largest circle, there's room for a lot of people in it.

Moving toward the center, the next circle includes people your teen may consider casual friends. Perhaps your son goes to the same parties or shares common friends with the people in this circle. Maybe your daughter is in several classes or on the soccer team with them. This circle is still fairly large, and its population probably shifts quite a bit, depending on circumstances.

The next circle is smaller yet and represents the people your teen considers friends. These are people your teen seeks out, whose opinions and feelings matter to her.

The innermost circle, closest to the center, includes those people closest to your teen. This is the privileged circle of intimacy. A true best friend would be found here. Very few people, male or female, ever earn this elite status.

Try This

Map out the circles of intimacy in your teen's life. Make a dark dot in the center of a sheet of paper. Draw four circles of increasing size around it. You probably won't to be able to list all of your teen's acquaintances and casual friends in the two outermost circles, but try to name a few. Next, write the names of your teen's friends in the second smallest circle. Now write the name or names of those special people in your teen's innermost circle. This is the person (or people) closest to your teen. Finally, place yourself and other family members where you think you belong in the circles of intimacy for your teen.

Were you able to list most of your teen's friends? How many of her closest friends do you know? Are there any holes in the list you'd like to fill? If so, you might go to your teen and tell her you did this exercise. Explain about the circles of intimacy, show her your work, and ask, "How did I do?" Then ask her to help you fill in any missing people.

Are you comfortable with the friendship choices she has made? If you are, you might say something like, "You seem to make really good choices when it comes to friends. That's not easy today, and you should be very proud of yourself. I know I'm proud of you." If you're concerned about some of your teen's friends, you might say, "I know and like a lot of your friends, but I don't know [name of friend] very well, and my impression is . . . ." Or "Maybe I'm wrong, but [name of friend] seems to be troubled . . . ." Then ask your teen how she feels about this person. Explain why you're concerned about your teen hanging out with this person or group. A word of caution: By speaking negatively about your teen's friends (and/or dates), you can easily cast yourself as the enemy and further unite your teen and this friend or group against you. So choose your words very carefully.

WHAT TO SAY?

If your teen has a friend you disapprove of, don't go to war. Instead, open the door to conversation. Guide your teen to make a thoughtful decision instead of forcing a decision on him.

Avoid saying . . .
"I forbid you to hang out with [name of person]. He's a bad influence. That's my final decision."

Instead, say . . .
"I want to learn more about your friendships. Tell me why hanging out with [name of person] matters to you."

If your teen says . . .
"I don't know. It just does."

You might say . . .
"What's it like to be with [name of person]?"

If your teen says . . .
"It's fun. It's exciting. [Name of person] is never boring, that's for sure."

You might say . . .
"Do you ever think there might be risks in hanging out with [name of person]?"

continued ⟶

If your teen says . . .
"Maybe."

You might say . . .
"What are your plans for dealing with those risks?"

By inviting conversation with this series of questions, you've learned more about your teen's friend. You've discovered something about why your teen is drawn to this person. You've helped him to acknowledge that the friendship might involve risks. You've encouraged him to plan ahead for times when it does. You've offered your support. Perhaps most important, you've guided him to look more closely at this particular friendship and reconsider it on his own.

Sometimes a teen chooses a friend simply because she likes the person. But sometimes a teen is friendly with someone because that person provides something she wants or needs—an "in" to the popular crowd or a particular clique, or even a ride to school. If a troublesome friendship seems to be based principally on serving specific needs for your teen, try to come up with other ways of meeting those needs. If your teen still holds onto this friendship, keep talking with her about your concerns. Be willing to either 1) set limits if your concerns are well-founded, or 2) admit you were wrong if they weren't, and allow for the fact that her taste in friends may be different from yours.

How difficult was it to figure out where you and other family members fit into the circles of intimacy? Are you where you'd like to be? If you are, great. If you aren't, you can do something about it. You might use the circles of intimacy exercise to talk with your teen about how that feels to you, and to ask how she feels. Sometimes the distance between you is due to some thing(s) you're doing. Ask your teen about this. Tell her that you want her honest answers. You might say, "I know you hate it when I do or say [give an example of something you know your teen doesn't like]. I'm trying to work on changing that. Please don't give up on me. I love you, and I want us to be close." If the distance is due to your teen, you might say, "I'd like to be closer to you. It makes it really hard when [give an example of something your teen does or says]." Or "It really hurts me that we aren't closer. Is there anything we can do together to help with that?" Follow these conversations with meaningful actions. Prove that you're willing to do your part to improve your relationship with her.

You might update your teen's intimacy circles every few months and see what happens. Do the names stay in the same place, or do they change? If you initially knew most of the people in your teen's life, don't get too confident.

Relationships change at all ages, but especially with teens. Revisiting this exercise can be a way of keeping your finger on the pulse of your teen's relationships. By showing a continued active interest in the people populating your teen's life, you're demonstrating that you care and want to be close.

Learn as much as you can about your teen's friends by listening to the stories she tells. By building a close relationship with your teen, you're increasing your chances of having a positive influence on her decisions about relationships and sexual behavior.

JUST THE FACTS

■ Peers have a great deal of influence over teens, and much of it is positive. For a girl, the more friends she has at low risk of pregnancy, the less her own risk of pregnancy becomes.[1]

■ In a national survey of teens, 80 percent said their decisions about sex and relationships are influenced by "what their parents have told them." When making decisions about sex and relationships, 79 percent weigh "what their parents might think."[2]

Dating

To encourage the sexual behavior patterns you'd like your teen to follow, what pattern of dating will you endorse? Do you want your teen to avoid all social contact with potential partners until a certain age? If so, what age? Why? When is it okay to go out with potential partners in groups? What about double dating? When is single dating okay? Will you encourage your teen to "play the field," or is it okay for him to be in an exclusive relationship? Do you think your positions on these issues will change as your teen gets older? Talk with him about your expectations and values. Explain why you feel as you do. Invite him to share his own feelings and values with you.

Some parents try to relive or improve on their own adolescence by living through their teens. If you went out every night of the weekend and twice on Sunday but your teen shows no interest in following suit, you may worry that he has a social problem. If you feel badly about not having been popular when you were younger, you may transfer your concern onto a perfectly contented teen. Try to remember: This is your teen's life, and he has his own needs and feelings, which may be very different from yours at his age.

Dating gives teens an opportunity to find out what they like and don't like in a partner. Dates are experiments—especially first dates. Encourage your teen to be open-minded about potential dates and to take some time before settling into an exclusive relationship.

SETTING LIMITS

Setting limits with children is never easy. With teens, it's especially challenging, because they're constantly seeking more independence and freedom. This is one of the developmental tasks of adolescence, and it's perfectly normal—if only it weren't so hard on parents.

Exactly when you allow a teen to start dating, in a group or individually, will be a personal decision based on your values. Some parents go strictly by age. Others have different guidelines for boys and girls. There is no magic formula, and each family and teen is different, but we do have some suggestions.

Don't be afraid to trust your values and instincts. If you think your teen is too young to go on a date, but she complains that everyone else is dating, you can say, "I'm sure their parents think it's okay, but I don't. I'm sorry if that makes you unhappy, but I can't agree to something I think is wrong." Then explain why. You might also explain what you feel is appropriate for your teen. For example, if you think one-on-one dating is not appropriate but group dating is, you could say, "I don't think that going out with just one person is okay for people your age. If you want to go out with a group, that's fine with me, as long as I know where you're going and who you're with." That information—where your child is and who she's with—is vital.

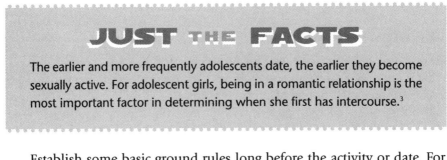

JUST THE FACTS

The earlier and more frequently adolescents date, the earlier they become sexually active. For adolescent girls, being in a romantic relationship is the most important factor in determining when she first has intercourse.[3]

Establish some basic ground rules long before the activity or date. For example, in addition to learning where she's going and who with, what time will she be home? What are her current plans? If her plans change, what do you expect her to do? Call you no matter what? Wait until she gets home and tell you then? The consequences of breaking rules should be in place and clearly understood before she walks out the door.*

Many teens object when their parents ask for details about their social life. They often feel they aren't being trusted, or that they're being treated like babies. Remain calm, but stand firm.

---

* For more on this topic, see "Reinforcement, Encouragement, Punishment, and Logical Consequences" on pages 90–92.

For example, your young teen announces that he's going to a friend's house. You ask, "Will his parents be there?" He says, "I don't know." You might say, "I'm sorry, but I don't think it's okay for kids your age to be at someone's house without a responsible adult around. Please find out if his parents will be there. If they won't be there, I can't let you go." Let your teen do the calling, asking, and reporting back to you. If you have any doubts about whether he's being truthful, tell him, then call the parents yourself.

If your teen protests, "Stop treating me like a baby!" you might say, "I'm sorry you feel I'm treating you like a baby, but that's not what I'm doing. I'm setting limits because I care about you and I want you to be safe." If your position is that he isn't allowed to go to a party without adult supervision, don't let his pleading change your mind. Say something like, "You know the rule. I understand that you're upset, but the rule is there for your protection."

If your teen insists, "You just don't trust me!" there are two possible answers. If you do trust your teen, you can say, "I'm sorry you feel that way, but I think I've demonstrated my trust in you." Then give an example or two. If you really don't trust your teen, chances are that he has given you reasons not to. Briefly describe a time when he compromised your trust. Then say, "Because of that, I'm having trouble trusting you." Explain that trust is something that is earned. Once lost, it is hard—but not impossible—to regain, but that takes time and effort. You might say, "I want to be able to trust you again. Following the rule we have about no parents, no parties is one way to help me with that."

What if your teen claims, "Nobody else's parents have a rule like that"? First, that's probably not true. But even if it is true, going along with the crowd isn't necessarily the best choice for you and your family. You might tell your teen, "Maybe they don't, but we do. We have the rule because we love you and we want you to be safe. That's more important to us than anything else." You won't make your teen happier, but you will give him a model of how not to give into peer pressure—at any age.

NO MEANS NO

One of the powerful myths of our culture is that when people say no, particularly in the heat of passion, they don't really mean it. This must be addressed directly when your teen begins to date.

Under no circumstances does no mean yes. It doesn't even mean maybe. No means *Hold It, Stop, Do Not Pass Go*—as any toddler can tell you. No is not a word to use as a tease or a come-on. It should not even be used in innocent games, like "No! No! Don't tickle me!" when what a teen really wants is to be tickled.

Teens need to understand that in a dating relationship, each partner has the right to be respected by the other. Each has the right not to be physically, emotionally, or sexually taken advantage of or abused. If one partner says no, the other must stop. It doesn't matter if the partners have had sex once before or 1,000 times before. No means no.

Have many conversations with your teen about the importance of saying no—clearly and firmly—only when she means it. Encourage her to make her own decisions. Sexual activity is not something she should have to be talked into. Also, sexual arousal is not an excuse for avoiding responsibility or forgetting to be respectful. Help your teen understand that each individual is accountable for his or her own sexual behavior.

You might tell your teen that one way to prevent acquaintance rape is to set limits before starting any sexual activity. Then both partners know in advance where things are going and where they're not.*

CONTROL AND VIOLENCE

Sometimes, in a dating relationship, one teen tries to control the other—through public insults, separating the partner from her group of friends, or having the partner frequently check in with him. We've even known teens whose partners have tried to tell them what they could and couldn't wear.

If you sense that your teen is on either side of a battle for control, ask about the relationship—both about what's actually happening and about how she feels. Explain that positive, healthy relationships require mutual trust and respect for each other's independence. It's never appropriate to insult someone you care about. It's okay and even necessary for partners to maintain other friendships. If constant checking-in is the issue, remind your teen that loving relationships are founded in trust. If your teen is not being trusted or is not trusting her partner, ask her to explore the reasons. If trust cannot be established, the relationship may need to end. Keep giving your teen the message that trying to control another person is not acceptable.

Social control is one serious problem many teens experience in their relationships. Violence is another. Both boys and girls use physical force against each other, from hitting and slapping to actual use of weapons. It's hard to tell how widespread the problem really is, because different studies and surveys ask about it in different ways. Both teenage boys and teenage girls report being victims of physical violence in relationships.[4]

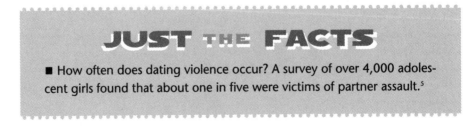

JUST THE FACTS

■ How often does dating violence occur? A survey of over 4,000 adolescent girls found that about one in five were victims of partner assault.[5]

---

* See "Dress Rehearsals" on pages 71–72 for an exercise that can help your teen learn to set limits.

■ A national survey found that one in eleven high school students said they had been hit, slapped, or physically hurt on purpose by their boyfriend or girlfriend in the past year.[6]

■ A study of eighth- and ninth-grade male and female students indicated that 25 percent had been victims of nonsexual dating violence, and 8 percent had been victims of sexual dating violence.[7]

Parents are often among the last to know that their teens are involved in violent relationships. Many teens who are victims of violence are too embarrassed—or too afraid—to talk about it. And parents seldom initiate discussions of dating violence with their teens. In one survey, only 8 percent of parents knew of any students at their teens' school who had been hit by someone they were dating. Only 36 percent of teens had had any discussion about dating violence with their parents.[8]

Your teen needs to hear from you about control and violence in dating relationships. Don't wait to hear from her, and don't assume that she already knows this information. Tell her exactly what you want her to do if she experiences control or violence in a dating relationship.*

DATING OLDER PEOPLE

Girls may be up to two-and-a-half years more socially advanced than boys their age. That's why some girls become interested in older guys. And older guys may be interested in girls who mature early. This can be appropriate, as long as the age difference is no greater than a year or two.

Dating someone more than a few years older can be a recipe for trouble. Teens who do this are more likely to get involved with drugs, alcohol, and sex.

JUST THE FACTS

■ The younger a girl is when she first has sexual intercourse, the greater the age difference is likely to be between her and her partner.[9]

■ Girls age seventeen and younger whose partners are more than three years older are significantly less likely to use contraception than their peers whose partners are closer in age.[10]

---

* For more on this topic, see "Abusive Relationships" on pages 114–115.

Don't be afraid to set age-related dating limits for your teen. You might say, "It's okay to have friends of different ages. But at this stage, it's not okay for you to date anyone who's a lot older or younger than you."

Imagine that your fifteen-year-old daughter is smitten with a nineteen-year-old boy. All she talks about is "him." If she's not on the phone with him, every waking moment is spent trying to persuade you to let her go out with him. He may even be a nice guy, but you know he's too old for her. She argues that she's more mature than the other kids her age, and that you're just trying to keep her from growing up. Your instincts say it's wrong, but you don't want to ruin your relationship with your daughter. What do you do?

Explain to your daughter (and her boyfriend, if you can) that the business of being fifteen is very different from the business of being nineteen. The main jobs of a fifteen-year-old are to do well in school and learn how to participate more fully in her family and community. The job of the nineteen-year-old will vary, depending on his life goals. He may be starting a career in the world of work. He may be pursuing his college education. Some nineteen-year-olds are ready to take on the responsibilities of parenthood; a fifteen-year-old isn't.

Ask your daughter to think back to when she was eleven. Can she recall the clothes she wore? Her favorite shoes? Would she wear them now? Of course she wouldn't, because she's grown—physically and emotionally—and changed in the four years since then. What she loved and thought was terrific at eleven is no longer cool or even cute. The same kinds of changes occur in the teen years. What seems wonderful now may not be so great a year or two from now.

You might tell your daughter, "You may be more mature than other kids your age. But the fact is, you're fifteen. Healthy relationships happen among people who are equals. Fifteen-year-olds and nineteen-year-olds are not equal."

It's not only girls who date older guys. Some guys prefer dating older girls. Among teenagers of both sexes (and any sexual orientation), a large age difference usually puts one partner at a disadvantage. Often, age means power.

Is It Love?

Once your teen begins to date, he will probably fall in love at some point . . . or at least think he has. It just happens. He develops an irresistible attraction for someone he might not even know, someone he's just met, someone who never seemed that interesting before, but now, wow! His heart is pounding, he feels a warm glow all over, everything seems magical, and everyone disappears except the two of them.

Many people have felt like this at one time or another—even parents. "Love at first sight" is a familiar theme in movies and television shows. It's been a favorite plot in literature for centuries; consider what happened when Romeo crashed Juliet's party.

When it hits, the feeling is very special. It's intense. It's pleasurable. It's energizing and exciting. But it isn't love. Not yet, anyway.

LOVE AND LIMERENCE

That passionate feeling has been called a "mad crush," "chemistry," "infatuation," and "having the hots for someone." The terms change with the times, but the intensity of the feeling—and the confusion it can bring—doesn't.

In her book *Love and Limerence: The Experience of Being in Love*, Dorothy Tennov coined the term "limerence" to describe the passionate attraction that is frequently mislabeled love—that knot in the pit of your stomach, that flush when you see or accidentally touch your special someone.

Limerence may or may not be reciprocal, and if the object of your limerence doesn't share your attraction, that may not make your feelings any less intense. While limerence can plant the seeds of love, more often than not it's fleeting.

Here's an analogy we frequently use in our practice: If you're going to light a fire in a fireplace, you usually start with lots of newspaper at the bottom. Then you add a layer of twigs. Finally, you place the big logs on top. When you strike the match, the newspaper catches first. It burns with an intense heat, but one that's over quickly. That's why it wouldn't do to fill the whole fireplace with paper. But if the fire is well-laid, the paper will burn just long enough to light the twigs. The twigs will burn a bit more slowly, perhaps allowing the logs to catch. The logs need a longer time to get started, but once they're burning, you have a lasting fire.

Limerence is like that newspaper fire—it's immediate and intense but can quickly burn itself out. Love is more like the burning logs. It takes preparation and time for it to catch and grow into a steady flame, but once it does, it can provide plenty of heat and warmth.

A relationship that begins in limerence can deepen into love or it can burn itself out. Love can also develop in relationships that initially don't involve limerence—relationships built on friendship or shared interests.

Unfortunately, many pop songs, TV programs, movies, and books present limerence as the ultimate model of romantic love. Two people, undeniable attraction, and opportunity instantly turn into a night of rapture and glorious sex (usually unprotected). So what if they don't know each other's names or are dating each other's best friends? They're in love, right? No, they're not.

Combine media pressure and peer influence with the qualities of adolescence—inexperience, hormones, mood swings, turmoil (emotional, social, and physical)—and you can see why teens are especially prone to confusing limerence with love. You can understand why they sometimes make choices based on sexual attraction rather than on a careful weighing of values and compatibility.

Still, teens can understand the difference between love and limerence, although you may prefer to use a more teen-friendly term (such as "infatuation," "crush," or "chemistry") when discussing it with your teen. You can explain that getting to know another person well takes time. You can say that to experience love, we need to see our partner as a whole person, complete with talents and wonderful qualities as well as less pleasing habits and flaws. In the heat of passion, we don't often see our partner at all. Instead, we're focused on an ideal and captivated by the moment.

There's nothing wrong with limerence, and a lot right with it. But when limerence is confused with love, problems and heartache can result. A teen may decide to bend or defy family rules, begin a sexual relationship, start a pregnancy, or marry long before he's ready.

JUST THE FACTS

In one national survey, sexually active teens were asked why they decided to have sex for the first time. The most common reason given was that they "had met the right person."[11]

Many teens want to wait to have a sexual relationship until they've met the right person. The problem is, teens may meet lots of people who seem "right." Meeting the right person is only *part* of the equation. Based on their values, is having sex the right thing to do? Is this the right time? Are these the right circumstances? Is this the right point in a relationship? Are they doing it for the right reasons?

Even if your teen is convinced that it's love, love itself is not enough. A cultural cliché tells us that "love can move mountains." Actually, earth-moving equipment will do a better job. This is a hard message for teens to hear, but it's an essential one. Love is just one ingredient among the many needed for a satisfying, long-term relationship. It may be a necessary ingredient, but it isn't a sufficient one. Other factors—including compatibility, shared goals, constructive communication patterns, and the ability to resolve conflict—should all come into the picture.

Help your teen understand that all relationships, just like friendships, should consist of mutual respect, honest communication, and the enjoyment of each other's company. Love, which by our definition is mutual, also requires knowledge and acceptance of yourself and your partner. The core of any true loving relationship is friendship, seasoned by experiencing tough as well as happy times together.

WHAT TO SAY?

Look for opportunities to discuss love and limerence, but keep in mind that many teens feel everything intensely. To some teens, a two-week relationship seems to last forever. Shared movie popcorn can symbolize commitment. A single long phone conversation or an instant message on a computer screen can confirm that a soul mate's been found. As a parent, you'll need to walk a fine line between helping your teen form realistic expectations and acknowledging that the adolescent's world of emotional relationships differs from the adult's.

If your teen says . . .
"I'm so in love with [name of person]."

You might say . . .
"It sounds like you're really attracted to him. That's a strong feeling, and a wonderful one, but do you think it's really love?"

If your teen says . . .
"I know it's love!"

You might say . . .
"Maybe it's limerence [or infatuation, or chemistry, or a crush, or whatever term you want to use]. What do you think?" Then talk about some of the differences between love and infatuation.

If your teen says . . .
"Tanya and James just had their three-week anniversary. They're totally in love."

You might say . . .
"That sounds like a special relationship. But do you think it's really love? Can people really love each other in three weeks? That may seem like forever, but it's not very long." Then talk about some of the reasons why love takes time to develop.

Talk with your teen about how his feelings for someone can change— even during a long-term committed relationship. Sometimes he'll feel friendship, sometimes limerence, and sometimes love. If his girlfriend has hurt his feelings, he may still care deeply for her but not like her much at the moment. Even people who are very close hurt each other, sometimes without meaning to. The closer you dance to your partner, the greater the risk of stepping on her toes. Ask your teen about his relationship, and ask what his feelings are.

Adolescence is a time of change and testing the waters. Teen relationships come in many varieties and intensities. Some last days, others months or even years. Some teens are cautious with their feelings, while others seem to fall in and out of limerence repeatedly. Some think that school, sports, or theater is more important than relationships, and others look to group activities as a safe way to "kind of" date, but without the pressure.

With your guidance and support, your teen can learn and appreciate the difference between limerence and love, and learn from his relationships—even the ones that don't turn out as he had hoped.

Breaking Up

A teen's romantic relationships can be extremely intense. The sense of closeness and the feeling of "you and me against the world," coupled with strong physical attraction and sheer exhilaration, can easily become the focus of her thoughts, conversations, and daydreams. It's natural for your teen to feel that she's found the love of her life and she'll never feel this way again.

If those strong feelings fade—and they often disappear as suddenly and mysteriously as they flared up—your teen may feel that she's fallen out of love. Take her feelings seriously. Try not to dismiss them as puppy love, especially if she's experiencing her first case of heartache. You can help her to accept a breakup she wasn't prepared for, or advise her on how to end a relationship gracefully.

If your teen is on the receiving end of a breakup, she may be convinced that she did something wrong, or she may think that if she had just one more chance, she could make her former partner love her again. Teens need to learn that feelings don't work like that. You can't make someone else feel something; you can only control yourself and your own feelings. Help her understand that if her former partner isn't interested in her anymore, she needs to let go.

If your teen doesn't come to you but you know there's something wrong, wait until you sense a time when she's more open. Approach her gently with something like, "It's obvious to me that you're hurting. I may not have the right answers, but I love you and want to be here for you any way I can. Talking sometimes helps." Or "It hurts me to see you hurt. Maybe talking about it could help."

Your teen might say that her boyfriend broke up with her and wonder aloud what she did wrong. Many concerned parents want to jump in and defend their teen—or even attack the ex-partner. Instead, wait and listen. Lead your teen to explore the specifics of the relationship and why she thinks it ended. Sometimes relationships end simply because they have run their course. Sometimes they end because one partner wants to move on. Sometimes they end because one partner did something "wrong," or something the other partner perceived as wrong. If the latter is the case with your teen's breakup, and she's blaming herself, remind her that nobody's perfect. We all mess up. That's part of what being a teen and dating are about—making mistakes and learning from them. You might want to give an example of how you, as a teen, made a similar mistake and learned from it.

Teens are often black-and-white in their thinking. Expect to hear words like *always* ("It's always going to feel this way"), *never* ("I never do anything right"), *everything* ("Everything I do is wrong"), and *nothing* ("Nothing ever goes right for me"). You might counter these statements by saying something like, "I'm sorry you feel that way, but I don't agree." Then give recent examples of things that did work out for her, or examples of how well she did at something.

WHAT TO SAY?

If you learn that your teen's girlfriend has just broken up with him, invite him to talk with you. Encourage him to share his feelings and his frustrations. Offer to just listen, if that's what he wants. Or ask if he'd like to hear any ideas or feedback from you.

If your teen says . . .
"I'm going to keep calling until she promises to see me again."

You might say . . .
"Maybe you can think about that for a minute. What if you were the one who broke up with her? Would you want her to keep calling you? How would that make you feel?"

If your teen says . . .
"It's all my fault. I messed up everything."

You might say . . .
"I know that you feel that way right now. I'm sorry that you're hurting. But it's not all your fault. It's hard for one person to make or break a relationship. It usually takes two. What can you learn from how you handled this relationship?"

If you know that your teen wants to break off a relationship, encourage her to do so with respect for the other person's feelings. If she puts off doing anything about it, ask her why. Maybe she's staying in the relationship because she feels sorry for her partner. Help her to understand that she must also be true to herself.

If your teen says . . .
"If Chris calls, tell him I'm not here."

continued ➝

You might say . . .
"I hope you're not really asking me to lie for you. I'm sorry, but I can't do that. Besides, you're going to have to talk to Chris sooner or later. Why not get it over with? If you want, you can practice on me. Pretend I'm Chris. What do you want to tell me?" Then help your teen come up with an honest but gentle way to talk with her soon-to-be-ex boyfriend.

If your teen says . . .
"I told Chris's friend Timothy to tell him that I don't want to go with him anymore."

You might say . . .
"I know you don't want to talk with Chris directly, and I understand why. It's going to be hard. It's going to hurt. But this is between you and Chris, don't you think? How would you feel if you were Chris? Would you want to hear the bad news from someone else?"

If your teen says . . .
"I don't love Chris anymore, but it'll hurt him if I break up with him."

You might say . . .
"I know you care for Chris and you don't want to hurt him. But is that a good reason to stay with him? What do you think?" Then help your teen develop a kind but firm way to explain that the relationship is over.

There's no getting around it: Breaking up is painful. At first, when the pain of rejection and sense of loss are most intense, your teen may feel as if her heart is literally broken. Be as supportive and empathetic as you can. Help her maintain her self-esteem by focusing on her strengths. Remind her that just because one boy doesn't like her doesn't mean she's not likable.

Your teen may feel that she doesn't want to mend. To imagine getting over a love she once cherished sounds cruel or heartless. How can love end?

Try This

To get in touch with what your teen may be feeling, think back on your first love. Chances are, that relationship ended long ago. Can you remember how you felt at the time? Can you reconnect with those feelings? You probably have a different perspective on them now.

We're not suggesting that you share this private memory, although you may want to let your teen know that you've felt emotional pain, too. A word of caution: Avoid saying or implying that you know what she's thinking or feeling. She's likely to respond, "You couldn't *possibly* know how I feel," and that's the end of your conversation. Instead, acknowledge that each person is unique. Tell your teen that you can only imagine what she's feeling. Then explain that attraction may diminish, the pain of separation may lessen, but love doesn't end. She may always carry a special feeling for that person in her heart, and that's not necessarily a bad thing.

Try to help your teen see that the end of a relationship doesn't mean she'll never find love again. As a parent, you know that love isn't a limited commodity—there's plenty to go around. But for a teen who's just experienced a painful breakup, this may not seem true. Your teen may be deeply hurt. Be compassionate and reassuring. Show her that you know she's unhappy and you're there for her. Let her know that even though it may not seem that way right now, you believe she'll eventually recover and form other satisfying relationships.

DEPRESSION

When a relationship ends, it's okay for your teen to grieve for the loss of a special person and the good times they shared. It's okay for him to feel sad. But when sadness becomes depression, teens need help. How can you tell if your teen is depressed? Here are some warning signs to watch for:[12]

- changes in eating habits (too much or too little)
- changes in sleeping patterns (too much or too little)
- low energy or constant fatigue
- withdrawal from social contact
- loss of interest in things he used to enjoy
- less attention to hygiene
- prolonged periods of irritability
- feelings of hopelessness
- loss of concentration
- falling grades and inattention to schoolwork and other responsibilities
- suicidal thoughts or gestures

What can you do if you think your teen might be heading toward depression? Ask him how he feels. Tell him you're there for him. Spend time with him. Invite him to talk, and listen when he does. Set firm but loving limits. For example, if your teen says, "I'll never go out again," you might say, "It's okay to feel that way. You can stay home this weekend if you really want to. But next Tuesday, there's no school; the family is going to the movies, and I expect you to join us."

Explain that pain is a part of life. There's no way around it. But sometimes we can choose the kind of pain we'll experience. If we choose to connect with others, we may get to feel love, passion, joy, warmth, and lots of other good things. But when a relationship ends, there will be the pain of loss. If we choose to disconnect emotionally, we may protect ourselves from the pain of loss, but we then have the pain of isolation and loneliness. Being emotionally disconnected hurts, too. This is a tough choice that even adults struggle with.

Real depression *is not* something that just goes away. It *is not* something that people snap out of on their own. It *is* treatable. If your teen doesn't show signs of recovering from the wounds of a broken relationship in a few weeks, seek professional help. Let him know that you won't give up and he will feel better.

One of the warning signs of depression listed above is "suicidal thoughts or gestures." These are some of the possible danger signs of suicide:[13]

- talking or joking about suicide
- statements about being reunited with a deceased loved one
- statements about hopelessness, helplessness, or worthlessness ("Life is useless," "Everyone would be better off without me," "It doesn't matter; I won't be around long anyway," "I wish I could just disappear")
- preoccupation with death (recurrent death themes in music, literature, or drawings)
- writing letters or leaving notes referring to death or "the end"
- suddenly seeming happier, calmer
- loss of interest in things one cared about
- unusual visiting or calling people one cares about; saying good-byes
- giving possessions away, making arrangements, setting one's affairs in order
- self-destructive behavior (alcohol/drug abuse, self-injury or mutilation, promiscuity)
- risk-taking behavior (reckless driving/excessive speeding; carelessness around bridges, cliffs, or balconies; walking in front of traffic)
- having several accidents resulting in injury; close calls or brushes with death
- obsession with guns or knives

If you notice any of these danger signs, or if you hear your teen (or any teen) talking generally about life not being worth living or specifically about suicide, take this very seriously. Get help *immediately.*

CRISIS HOTLINES

1-800-SUICIDE
(1-800-784-2433)

The National Hopeline Network is for people who are depressed or suicidal, or those who are concerned about someone they love. It connects callers automatically to the nearest certified Crisis Center, where trained counselors answer calls 24 hours a day, 7 days a week. The Network uses the ANI (Automatic Number Identification) system to route calls. If the nearest Crisis Center is at maximum volume, the call is immediately rerouted to the next closest center. People in crisis usually reach a trained counselor within two to three rings, or about 20 to 30 seconds, from the moment they dial 1-800-SUICIDE. Callers should never encounter a busy signal or voicemail. For more information, visit the Web site at *www.hopeline.com.*

1-800-621-4000

This toll-free number is the 24-hour hotline of the National Runaway Switchboard, a not-for-profit volunteer organization whose mission is to provide confidential crisis intervention and referrals to youth and their families. They deal with all kinds of adolescent problems, including teen depression and suicide. They can help you or your teen connect with counseling services in your area. For more information, visit the Web site at *www.nrscrisisline.org.*

1-800-999-9999

The Covenant House Nineline provides immediate crisis intervention, support, and referrals for runaways, abandoned youth, and those who are suicidal or in crisis. Help is available for children, teens, and adults. For more information, visit the Web site at *www.covenanthouse.org.*

1-800-448-3000

The Girls and Boys Town National Hotline is a crisis hotline teens can call 24 hours a day. A professional counselor will listen and offer advice on any issue (depression, suicide, identity struggles, family troubles, and other problems). For more information, visit the Web site at *www.girlsandboystown.org.*

CHOOSE YOUR MODEL AND CUSTOMIZE IT

In our chocolate-loving family, we have a number of recipes for chocolate-chip cookies and brownies. While each is a little different, they all have one thing in common: No nuts in anything, no matter what the recipe says. Your family may enjoy all kinds of exotic nuts blended into their desserts, but not the Mirons.

Choosing a model of sexuality education for your teen is like selecting and then customizing a favorite recipe. What works for one family may not work for another. We can't tell you what's right for you and your teen. But we can suggest three basic models—abstinence, delayed sexual expression, and responsible sexual involvement—and put them within a context of related issues that may affect your decision about which one to choose.

The Interpersonal Toolbox

Regardless of what your family's approach to sexuality may be, certain relationship skills are essential for anyone who's going to make good sexual decisions. These include respect, integrity, assertiveness, and love.

RESPECT

Two necessary ingredients of a positive, healthy sexual relationship are a strong sense of self-respect and respect for others. When teens don't feel good about themselves, they're more likely to give in to peer pressure or use sexual activity to gain popularity or acceptance.

The best way to ensure that your teen will march to her own drum (and preferably to a rhythm you approve of) is to help her build her self-esteem. Encourage and recognize her for her accomplishments, strengths, contributions, and self-initiated activities. Applaud her unique qualities. When you notice her acting responsibly, acknowledge and reinforce her behavior.

Help her understand that it's okay to be wrong. When she makes a mistake or an unwise decision, criticize the act, not the teen. Remember that nobody's perfect. When you make a mistake, admit it.

Guide her to respect others. Model respect for others in your own behavior. It's not okay to tell or laugh at jokes that target individuals or groups based on their race, religion, ethnic background, or sexual orientation. Point out that people who put others down are acting out of insecurity or ignorance. Reinforce the idea that people are different, and that differences don't make us better or worse. How does this relate to sexual behavior? For your teen to be able to make decisions that go against the majority, she needs to see differences as acceptable and valuable.

INTEGRITY

Integrity is doing the right thing just because it's the right thing to do. Help your teen learn the importance of following through on commitments to himself and others. Let him know that if he doesn't keep his promises—even if he's the only one who knows it—he undermines his personal integrity.

If your teen says he'll walk the dog, make it clear that you expect him to do it. If he makes plans with one friend and then gets a call from another, encourage him to honor the original commitment, even if the second invitation is more appealing. If he vows to cut down on junk food, help him understand that he loses integrity in his own eyes if he eats a whole bag of chips at one sitting. Learning to honor small commitments lays the foundation he'll need to follow through on the big ones, such as a decision to refrain from sexual activity or to be sexually responsible.

ASSERTIVENESS

Many teens only have two styles of communication in their toolbox. Either they're passive and give in to others, or they're aggressive and try to dominate them. Being passive is the teen's Child or Adolescent saying, "I don't count for much, so whatever you want goes." Being aggressive is the Child or Adolescent saying, "You don't count for much, so we'll do what I want."*

A third and more valuable tool is assertiveness—a position of mutual respect that implies, "I count, and so do you." An assertive teen's response to sexual pressure is, "You can want to have sexual intercourse as a way of showing that you love me. I can love you and not want to have sexual intercourse."

Teens need to practice assertiveness, starting with little things. If your teen orders iced tea at a restaurant and the server brings her soda, encourage her to politely point out the mistake and ask that the server bring her iced tea. Learning to handle situations assertively will build her confidence. Eventually, when she's pressured to engage in a sexual activity she's not comfortable with or ready for, she'll be able to look her partner in the eye and say no assertively.**

---

* See "The Miron Model" on pages 19–27.
** "Dress Rehearsals" on pages 71–72 can help your teen build assertiveness skills.

LOVE

Before they can make sound sexual decisions, teens need to know what love is—and isn't. It's hard for your teen to maintain his bearings and commitments when he's being swept up by intense infatuations and hormones. Having a strong set of personal values is essential. So is understanding the difference between short-term physical attraction and long-term feelings of love.*

Help your teen learn to identify and express his own feelings. Model empathy—the ability to recognize and understand the feelings of others. Make your home a place where all family members are free to talk about their feelings.

Topics and Influences

As professional sex therapists and educators with children of our own, we believe that a teen's sexuality education should include current, factual information about birth control, safer sex, and sexual pleasure.** Teens also need to know how alcohol, drugs, and other influences can affect their sexual decision making.

ALCOHOL AND DRUGS

Alcohol and drugs can impair judgment, and sexual decisions are often made under their influence. Many teens report that they were drinking when they first had sexual intercourse. We once saw a bumper sticker that said, "If you drink, don't park—accidents cause people."

It's not only sexual activity that's affected when teens use alcohol and drugs. Teens who drink are more likely to engage in verbally and physically aggressive behavior with a partner.[1]

All teens should learn the facts about alcohol and drugs. "Just say no" isn't enough. Teens will ultimately decide for themselves whether to abstain from, use, or abuse these substances. To make positive, healthy decisions, they need solid information, not slogans. They also need to know their parents' values about alcohol and drug use.

Talk with your teen about why you feel she should not use alcohol and drugs. Make sure she knows your local and state laws related to teen alcohol and drug use. If you use alcohol, model responsible behavior.

Ask your teen what drugs she has been exposed to and where. At school? At parties? In the park? On the street? Ask her if other kids she knows are using drugs. (You'll probably get a more honest answer if you keep this question general instead of asking about specific friends.) To learn more about how prevalent drugs are in her life, you might ask, "If you wanted to use [name

---

* See "Is It Love?" on pages 50–51.

** See "Issue 5: Safer Sex" (pages 170–205) and "Issue 6: Sexual Pleasure" (pages 206–217).

of a specific drug], would you know how and where to get it?" Help her practice ways to resist peer pressure to experiment with alcohol and drugs.*

JUST THE FACTS

■ About one-quarter of sexually active ninth- through twelfth-grade students report using alcohol or drugs during their most recent sexual encounter.[2]

■ In one study of unplanned pregnancies in fourteen- through twenty-one-year-olds, one-third of the girls who had gotten pregnant had been drinking when they had sex. Ninety-one percent of them reported that the sex was unplanned.[3]

■ Boys who drink or smoke at a young age are 40 percent more likely to start having sex than boys who don't drink or smoke. For girls, that figure jumps to 80 percent.[4]

■ Thirteen percent of teens say that they've done something sexual while using alcohol or drugs that they might not have done if they were sober.[5]

POPULAR CULTURE

Today's teens live in a multimedia world. That world sends many messages about romance and sexuality that are often at odds with reality, and also with what most parents would like their teens to believe. Buy these jeans and you'll be sexy. Try that fragrance and your partner will melt with desire. Dress and act like this teen idol and you'll be cool, too.

How can parents counter these messages? Some parents worry that their teens will think their opinions are old-fashioned or irrelevant. Others withhold their comments because they don't want to hear the usual "Oh, Mom!" or "Oh, Dad!"

When our daughters were much younger, a popular song aired on the radio several times a day. It spoke to a set of values that was the exact opposite of ours. At first, we weren't sure what the lyrics were saying, so we asked our daughters about them. Once we understood the lyrics, we began a discussion of why we liked the artist, loved the melody—and hated the words.

We got the "Oh, Mom, Dad, it's only a song" response, but our kids also heard our side—that we didn't care if it was only a song, we strongly disagreed with what it was saying. We explained that while the song emphasized

---

* "Dress Rehearsals" on pages 71–72 can help your teen build resistance skills.

the importance of money and possessions, we believe in the importance of things like kindness and honesty. Then we asked our daughters what they thought. They liked the music, loved the artist—and thought the words were dumb and wrong.

When you hear a song that contradicts your values, talk with your teen. Ask him what he thinks. When you see a music performer or video advertising sexual messages, directly or through innuendo, start a dialogue about it. Invite your teen's point of view. Listen. Share yours without lecturing or preaching. Make sure it's a two-way conversation. You may not agree on everything, but you'll probably find some common ground.

PEERS

One of the main tasks of adolescence is to establish an identity as an individual apart from the family. Instead of seeking approval from parents, some teens seek it from their peers. A teen's sexuality decisions may be strongly influenced by peer pressure.

In the world of the adolescent, sex is a major topic. It's probably on your teen's mind much of the time. Most of his friends are talking about it. And the statistics indicate that many of his peers are doing more than talking.

Some teens are embarrassed about being virgins. When other kids boast about their sexual adventures, they feel inadequate or left out. They may wonder if something is wrong with them.

Help your teen understand that at least some of the sexual boasting he hears is just talk. Some of his peers may be inventing or exaggerating their sexual exploits to make themselves seem more important and experienced. Even if they're telling the truth, everyone is different. Sexual values and decisions are an individual thing. What's right for one person may not be right for another.

If your teen chooses not to engage in sexual activity, he may be excluded and called names—dork, baby, prude, goody-goody, queer. Remember that ridicule from one's peers hurts. It's not easy to stand up for your beliefs among people whose acceptance is important to you.

Not all peer pressure is bad, though, and not all teens make unhealthy decisions. Teens often support each other through difficult times. Many rally around causes that promote sexual wellness and positive relationship values. One group of teens we know developed an outreach program to educate their peers about the human immunodeficiency virus (HIV, the cause of AIDS). Another offered peer counseling in their high school. As adults, we should recognize and encourage the inner strength and resources of our teens.

Your teen's best defense against negative peer pressure is a clear understanding of his own beliefs. It's easy to influence someone who's uncertain or who hasn't given any thought to an issue. It's much harder to influence someone who knows his own mind.

AUTHORITY FIGURES

You may feel that your influence over your teen is slipping away. In fact, you're still an important authority figure in her life. She cares what you think and believe, even if she doesn't always let you know. That's why we keep encouraging you to talk with your teen. But while talk is important, actions speak louder than words.

Teens learn a lot from the behavior they observe. If you don't want your teen to smoke cigarettes but you're a smoker, what message are you sending? When you drive, do you obey the speed limits? Do you follow the rules and laws in your community? If you use alcohol, do you drink responsibly? What about drugs—prescription, over-the-counter, and other kinds? How do you talk about your boss? If you're the boss, how do you talk about and behave toward your employees? How do you interact with religious leaders, your teen's teachers, neighbors, and other family members? How do you treat your partner? How do you treat your teen? If you're separated or divorced from your teen's other parent, how do you relate to him or her? Do you handle conflict constructively? Do you respect authority?

What kind of role model are you? If you want your teen to adhere to certain values, the best way to communicate this is by your actions.

Your teen will encounter and be influenced by many other authority figures: teachers, coaches, older siblings and other family members, religious leaders, youth leaders, mentors. While you can hope that all will be positive role models, that's probably wishful thinking. Not all adults are fair, reasonable, or responsible in their approach to relationships. Some authority figures who are adored by teens may not reflect your values and beliefs. Your teen may idolize a student teacher who has multiple piercings, a tongue stud, and tattoos—body art you find unacceptable. What can you do? Probably not much. What can you say? A lot.

Learn as much as you can about the authority figures in your teen's life. Who does your teen like and dislike, and why? Offer your views on the ones you both know. See if you can distinguish those who've developed into Adults from those who haven't. When you see a teacher who models a quality you admire, point that out to your teen. For example, you might say, "I really like that your science teacher is teaching you about viruses and sexually transmitted infections. What's it like to be in her class? How do you feel about her?" When your teen complains about a teacher who uses power unfairly, talk with her about how that feels. Then, when you notice your teen using her power over a younger sibling, remind her of your earlier conversation. Tell her that she's a role model, too.

The sexuality and relationship messages coming from faith communities may or may not coincide with your values. Reinforce the beliefs you'd like your teen to adopt. If you disagree with certain positions, explain why.

If you believe that a grounding in your religion will help your teen with her sexual decision making, encourage her participation. If a sermon goes against some of your beliefs, or a religious leader advocates something you don't agree with, talk about it with your teen.

Authority figures also grow out of the popular culture. Companies pay fortunes to have well-known superstars advertise their products. These people have influence, but what messages are they sending your teen? Sometimes they're generous with their time and money, donating them to worthy causes. Point that out to your teen. You could even have fun with this and ask, "What if you were rich and famous? What would you do to make the world a better place?" or "What kind of messages would you try to give teens if you were a star?"

Sometimes superstars behave in ways that you don't approve of. Point that out, too. Don't be silent when you hear that a sports hero threw a tantrum on the court, or an unmarried movie star had a baby. You might say something like, "I don't care how talented he is; I think behaving like that is wrong," or "I don't care how rich and famous she is; I believe that people should wait until they're married to have babies." Ask your teen how she feels.

Older teens may also influence your teen's decisions about sexual expression and relationships. Sometimes they represent models of behavior you agree with. Other times, they don't. Either is an opportunity for you to talk with your teen. Despite the many other people your teen interacts with or observes, you're probably still the most important authority figure in her life.

JUST THE FACTS

Among teens ages fifteen through seventeen who had *not* had sexual intercourse, 64 percent said the main reason was worry about what their parents would think. Only 15 percent said the main reason was worry about what their friends would think.[6]

What Do You Want Your Teen to Do— or Not Do?

What sexual behaviors are—and are not—acceptable for your teen? Do you believe that sexual intercourse before marriage is permissible, but only within a committed relationship? Would you condone casual or recreational sex? Do you want your teen to abstain from sexual intercourse until marriage? If so, what exactly do you mean by "abstain"?

Write down your definition of the word *abstinence*. Ask your partner or other important adult(s) in your teen's life to do the same—stepparents, grandparents, aunts and uncles. Compare your definitions. Are they similar or very different? Are you surprised? Why or why not?

Does your definition simply mean abstinence from sexual intercourse? If so, how do you feel about other forms of shared sex? Does your definition allow for dry kissing? Wet kissing? Genital touching? Oral sex? Anal sex?* What do you really want your teen to abstain from?

If you feel that teens should not have sexual intercourse, are there any acceptable alternatives? Or do you believe that your teen must remain sexually inactive (celibate) until such time as your value system allows for full sexual expression? If you want your teen to abstain from any form of sexual gratification with others, do your values permit you to give her a positive message about masturbation? If the other people involved in raising your teen don't agree on these issues, how will you handle your differences?

This is not a test. There are no right or wrong answers, and you don't have to answer all the questions right away. But you'll want to keep them in mind as you choose a sexuality education model for your teen.

THE ABSTINENCE MODEL

Abstinence generally means not engaging in sexual intercourse (and possibly other forms of sexual activity) until marriage. Since it usually doesn't mean lifelong abstinence, but simply delaying intercourse until marriage, abstinence is actually a variation of the delay model, and within it are further variations. Some parents want their teens not to engage in any shared sexual activity. Others will accept some sexual contact with a partner, as long as it stops short of sexual intercourse.

Even if your teen is committed to abstaining from sexual intercourse until marriage, he will probably engage in some sexual experimentation in his teen years. You'll need to clarify for yourself and your teen what forms of shared sexual behavior are acceptable under your definition of abstinence. When you talk to your teen about abstinence, be specific about what you do and don't want him to do.

If your values permit it, offer positive messages about masturbation. If you want your teen to avoid shared sex, masturbation can be a healthy way to deal with sexual tension. You might say, "You'll hear lots of jokes about

---

* See "Issue 4: Sexual Expression" (pages 155–169).

masturbation, but the truth is, it's a safe way to learn about your body." Or "You know that our family doesn't believe in teens having oral sex or sexual intercourse, but masturbation is a safe way to ease sexual tension."

ABSTINENCE, NOT IGNORANCE

Speaking as sex therapists, educators, and parents, we strongly believe that abstinence shouldn't mean ignorance. If you want your teen to remain abstinent (however you define it) until marriage, she still should know the facts about sex and sexuality. Eventually, she will become sexually active, and she'll need to be well-informed. Giving your teen information before she needs it helps her build confidence and normalizes discussions about sex.

When you talk with your teen about sex, you're not only providing her with valuable information. You're also sending two important messages: that it's okay to talk about sex, and it's okay to talk about sex with *you*. Because of your willingness to share information, your teen will be as knowledgeable as her friends (or more knowledgeable) when they discuss sexual issues (which they will). And if, for whatever reason, your teen's resolve to be abstinent changes, she will be able to protect herself from sexually transmitted infections (STIs) and pregnancy.

Your abstinent teen will be exposed to all kinds of sexual messages as well as opportunities. If you want her to make positive, healthy decisions about her own behavior, she needs real information to base them on. Many teens who decide not to have sexual intercourse engage in other activities. For example, they don't equate oral sex with sex. But it is a form of sexual activity, and it can lead to STIs. By giving your teen sexuality information, you can help keep her safe while creating an environment that establishes you, the parent, as an available resource.

Some churches and youth groups organize abstinence campaigns and public pledges of virginity. The support of a group can be useful to teens who are wrestling with those issues. *Tip:* It's never "too late" to be abstinent. Teens who are sexually active can choose to stop.

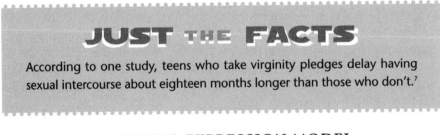

JUST the FACTS

According to one study, teens who take virginity pledges delay having sexual intercourse about eighteen months longer than those who don't.[7]

THE DELAYED SEXUAL EXPRESSION MODEL

Delaying sexual expression means waiting until certain conditions other than marriage have been met. These conditions vary, but they usually involve reaching a certain age or degree of commitment in a relationship;

passing some social landmark, such as high school or college graduation; or gaining financial independence.

If you choose any variation of this model, you'll need to give your teen the same tools and information you'd provide if you were asking him to remain abstinent. Specify the conditions under which your family feels various forms of sexual expression are acceptable, and explain your reasons for wanting him to meet those conditions.

THE RESPONSIBLE SEXUAL INVOLVEMENT MODEL

This model stresses that whenever a teen is involved in sexual activity, she should participate safely. The emphasis here is on *how* a teen will engage in sexual behavior rather than *when* or under what conditions.

Many parents who choose this model recognize that their teen may become sexually active regardless of whether they approve, and they want their teen to behave in a sexually responsible way. These parents feel it's their job to give their teens the knowledge and skills they need to do this. If this model fits your values and goals, your discussions with your teen may focus on the emotional consequences and responsibilities of sexual choices.

Helping Your Teen Make Sexual Decisions

Guide your teen to develop a personal code of ethics to follow when making all kinds of decisions, including sexual decisions. Start by helping her articulate the values your family believes in.

Try This

Draw a picture of a shield. Ask your teen to imagine that, just like the knights in the days of King Arthur, your family is about to go into battle against an army of invaders. All the members of your family will need shields to protect them. In the past, shields were decorated with symbols of the knights' beliefs. For example, if a knight valued strength in battle, he might have a lion on his shield. If he valued education, he might have a book. Ask your teen to draw your family's shield, including images of the things your family stands for.

After your teen has created a family shield, invite her to create her own personal shield. This can be a starting point for a discussion of her values and beliefs. Listen closely to what she says, and remember that you don't have to agree.

In one family we worked with, the teen jumped at the chance to draw his own shield. He started by drawing a dollar sign in the center, then drew dollar signs in each of the corners. When asked to explain the meaning of his shield, he said he felt that money was the most important thing in life. It could protect him from just about anything. He even pointed to a famous person he felt had gotten away with murder because the person had enough money to pay for good attorneys. His parents had no idea that he felt this way, and they were able to use this exercise to explore their own very different opinions.

Encourage your teen to think about things she believes would give her moral integrity and help her feel good about herself. Ask if she's willing to share her sexual code of ethics with you. What does she believe is sexually right or wrong? What does she want to do, and what does she want to avoid?

Suggest that she develop a personal position on issues like the role of love in sexual behavior, when and whether it's right to engage in various sexual activities, premarital sexual intercourse, sexual boundaries, condoms, birth control, and abortion, to name a few. She can write her position on a piece of paper or in a journal. She can share it with you or keep it private. You might tell your teen that in some ways, she's like a knight of the Round Table. She may not fight with a sword, but she will come in contact with people, young and old, who will attack what she stands for. Her position will be her shield.

Try This

Do this exercise with your teen. Each of you will need a piece of paper. Draw a line down the center. In the left-hand column, list all of the reasons for postponing sexual activities or intercourse that you can think of. In the right-hand column, list reasons for *not* waiting. Afterward, compare and discuss your lists. What are the similarities? The differences?

When differences arise (as they almost certainly will), try not to let your Child or Adolescent blurt out, "How could you think that?" Instead, your Adult might calmly say, "I don't understand your reasoning. Could you please explain it to me and help me understand why you feel that way?"

Here are some of the responses that teens have shared with us.

Reasons to Wait	Reasons Not to Wait
• don't want to have a baby	• to get love
• might get HIV/AIDS	• all my friends are doing it
• want to finish school first	• nobody tells me what to do

Reasons to Wait	Reasons Not to Wait
• it hurts	• to show love
• my parents might find out	• to keep my girlfriend/boyfriend
• want to wait for marriage	• curiosity
• too young	• to get even with my parents
• it's a sin	• to get even with an old girlfriend/boyfriend
• would get a bad reputation	• in a serious relationship, it's natural
• waiting for the right person	
• my religion says to wait	• ready to experiment
• not ready yet	• to be grown-up
• afraid	• it feels good
• don't want to get a sexually transmitted infection	• in love
	• to get a baby—someone who will love me forever

Once your teen has developed his own sexual code of ethics and explored his own reasons to postpone or engage in sexual activities, talk more about how a relationship requires two active partners. Remind your teen that he's responsible for his own behavior, and also for letting his partner know where he stands on sexual issues. Encourage him not to leave it up to his partner to guess where his boundaries are. Tell him to be strong and not to let anyone impose different values on him.

DRESS REHEARSALS

Broadway producers and directors know that no matter how many times they go over a script, the actual performance is a very different experience. The music may not start on cue. The leading lady's costume may be too tight for her to run across the stage. That's why they have dress rehearsals to simulate the conditions of opening night.

In the confusing, highly charged world of growing up, sexual decisions are frequently unrehearsed. They're made onstage, under the influence of peer pressure, often mixed with alcohol and drugs.

To help your teen avoid sexual activity she doesn't want to engage in, take a cue from the theater and rehearse situations that may be difficult for her. Following are some sample lines and responses to get you started. Your job is to help your teen work out her own responses to the lines. This is a proactive way to prepare your teen for many challenges she might face.

Have fun with this. Be creative. Ask your teen to make up her own lines and responses. Tell her that she doesn't always have to give a reason—that saying "Because I don't want to" can be enough. Return to this exercise from time to time and explore new situations.

Tip: Even when rehearsing possible lines and responses with your teen, you probably won't feel comfortable saying, "If you love me, you'll have sex with me." Instead, phrase each line as a "what-if." Example: "What if someone told you, 'If you love me, you'll have sex with me'? What would you say back?"

Lines	Responses
"Everybody else is having sex. Why can't we?"	"I'm not everybody else. I'm me." OR "I don't believe everybody else is having sex. Even if they are, I don't care."
"If you love me, you'll have sex with me."	"If you love me, you'll respect my feelings."
"Look at this cool porn site I found on the Web."	"No, thanks. I don't want to."
"Why won't you give me a blow job? You can't get pregnant."	"Because I don't want to."
"I can't believe you won't even drink a beer. It's not like it's weed or something."	"I'm having a good time without alcohol."

Here are more lines you can cast as "what-ifs" and practice with your teen. Help her come up with appropriate responses—ones that match her values and beliefs.

- "If you won't have sex with me, I'm breaking up with you."
- "Do I look like I have a disease? Why do you want me to wear a condom? Don't you trust me?"
- "Come on, grow up. You can't stay a kid forever."
- "Don't you want to try it and find out what it's like?"
- "I don't have a condom with me."
- "You've got me so turned on I can't stop now."
- "I hate condoms. By the time you get it on, the mood's gone. I'll pull out in time."
- "You're on the pill, so why do I have to wear a condom?"
- "What's the matter with you? Are you frigid or something?"
- "If you get pregnant, I'll marry you."
- "We've had sex before. What's the problem now?"
- "I've got some good weed. Let's get high."

Sex and the Teen with Special Needs

Adolescence signals the dawn of sexual identity for all teens, including those who are emotionally, physically, or mentally challenged. They experience sexual feelings, thoughts, and arousal, and they need sexual information, support, and guidance.

The ostrich solution—sticking your head in the sand and pretending the issue isn't there—won't work. Not dealing with the issue suggests to your child that you think he is nonsexual or incapable of sexual relationships.

If you're the parent of a teen with special needs, your first task is to foster his self-acceptance and self-esteem. The normal self-consciousness of adolescence—the obsession with appearance, the constant comparisons between himself and his peers or between his own body and some imagined ideal—is likely to be even more traumatic for him.

Help your teen explore ways of expressing his sexuality regardless of his limitations. If your teen chooses to be sexually expressive with a partner, he'll need all the information that other teens need, and then some. Literature and support groups dealing with specific disabilities and conditions can offer invaluable help and support. Consult your physician or check out the possibilities on the Internet or at your library.

Whatever the challenge your teen faces—emotional, physical, mental, or a combination of all three—remember that sexuality is a natural part of everyone's life.

Sex Education in School

Most public schools in the United States teach some form of sex education. At the time of this writing, many use an abstinence-until-marriage program.

Abstinence-only education teaches that sexual activity outside of marriage is likely to have harmful psychological and physical effects. Critics of such programs—including the American Medical Association, Office of National AIDS Policy, National Institutes of Health, and the American Academy of Pediatrics—maintain there is no proof that abstinence-only sex education is effective in delaying the onset of intercourse. These organizations all support comprehensive sexuality education, including access to information on contraception and condoms.

In September 2000, the Kaiser Family Foundation, a nonprofit independent national health care philanthropy, released a report called *Sex Education in America: A View from Inside the Nation's Classrooms.** The report

---

* If you'd like to read the full report, call the foundation's publication request line at 1-800-656-4533 and ask for a free copy of publication #3048. The report is also available online at the foundation's Web site: *www.kff.org.*

was based on a series of national surveys of more than 4,000 public secondary school students and their parents, sex education teachers, and principals. Some of the study's findings include:[8]

- There are gaps between what parents want schools to teach and what is actually being covered in the classroom. Examples:
  - Ninety-seven percent of parents want their children to know what to do if a friend has been raped or assaulted. But only 59 percent of students say that topic was covered in their most recent sex education course.
  - Ninety-four percent of parents want their children to know how to deal with pressure to have sex. Seventy-nine percent of students say that topic was covered in their most recent sex education course.
  - Ninety-two percent of parents want their children to know how to get tested for HIV/AIDS and other STIs. Sixty-nine percent of students say that topic was covered in their most recent sex education course.
- Both parents and educators think that more time should be spent on sex education.
- Most parents surveyed want school sex education classes to cover more topics including condom usage, abortion, and sexual orientation.
- Some classes described as "abstinence-only" offer practical information about birth control and/or safer sex.
- Some classes described as "comprehensive" don't provide information about how to use contraceptives or where to get them.

Find out what your teen is—and isn't—learning in school. If some of the topics you feel should be addressed aren't being covered, make your voice heard. Most schools' programs inform parents of the content of their sex education programs. If you haven't been notified, ask the sex education teacher or school principal about the curriculum.

If you'd like to volunteer your time, energy, or knowledge to help teens learn accurate, appropriate sexual information, consult with sex educators in your community. You may be able to get involved in existing programs or be instrumental in starting new ones. *

---

* See "Resources" (pages 228–238) for many excellent sources of sexuality information.

WHAT DO TEENS WANT TO KNOW?

According to *Sex Education in America: A View from Inside the Nation's Classrooms,* these are the Top 10 topics students say they need more information about:

1. What to do in cases of rape or sexual assault
2. How to get tested for HIV and other sexually transmitted diseases (STDs)
3. STDs other than HIV/AIDS
4. HIV/AIDS
5. How to talk with a partner about birth control and STDs
6. How to deal with emotional consequences of being sexually active
7. How to talk with parents about sex and relationships
8. Birth control
9. How to deal with pressure to have sex
10. How to use and where to get birth control

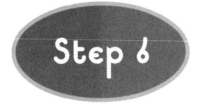

TALK WITH YOUR TEEN

A client we'll call David told us the following story: One day, when he was about six or seven years old and starting to ask questions about where babies come from, he and his younger sister were summoned to their parents' bedroom. His father closed the door. Since there was no one else in the house but the family dog, David thought this was odd.

A handful of pamphlets and charts materialized out of the nightstand drawer, and his parents launched into a detailed explanation of male and female anatomy and biology. To David, it seemed to go on forever, though it probably lasted about an hour. He recalls being vaguely embarrassed but mostly bored. He asked a few simple questions, but the answers he got were long-winded and not particularly helpful.

Among children who get any formal sexual education from their parents at all, David's experience is fairly typical. At some point, the parents deliver a one-time lecture about the birds and the bees.

Even if you haven't yet given your child the birds-and-the-bees talk, you've been educating him since birth in such aspects of sexuality and relationships as touching and affection. You've changed his diapers, kissed his boo-boos, and felt his fevered brow. You've held his hand while crossing the street and held his seat as he learned to ride a bike. You've probably rubbed, patted, and tickled his back and tummy. And he's learned by watching you relate to your partner or other adults.

The point is: You're already a pro at the informal sex education of your child. When you talk with your teen about love, relationships, and sex, it might feel more formal, and in some ways it will be. But it's really a variation on something you already know how to do.

Try This

Think about some of the ways you've educated your teen about touching and affection throughout his life. How have you taught him the

continued ➝

difference between touching that's okay and touching that's not okay? What messages, direct or indirect, have you given him about affection? Did you cuddle with him while reading or watching TV? Did you give and accept hugs? Hold his hand? Kiss him goodnight? Did you kiss your partner hello? Good-bye? Goodnight? How did you react when your teen was younger and behaved aggressively toward other people?

Setting the Stage

When parents imagine talking with their children about love, relationships, and sex, they often think this will occur under ideal conditions. They'll have the time to prepare and present a logical, convincing case for the model of sexual behavior they want their teens to follow—when the right time comes.

If teaching sexuality were like teaching chess, that might work. You could store the chess set in the attic so your toddler wouldn't gnaw on the pieces or lose them. Later, when your child seemed ready to learn the rules of the game, you could retrieve the pieces from the safety of their storage place and begin teaching.

But teaching sexuality is more like playing a video game. You're reacting to a constantly changing screen. And just when you think you've mastered the game, you're pushed to the next level of difficulty.

When is the "right time" for a child to learn "the facts of life"? Many parents wonder about this. There's no simple answer, but here's a good rule of thumb: If a child is old enough to ask the question, she's ready to hear the answer.

This doesn't mean that David was ready for a crash course on human biology and reproduction. Let's give his parents credit; at least they didn't tell him that babies come from the cabbage patch or are delivered by storks. What kind of answer would have satisfied him? It's hard to tell at this distance. But it might have been enough if his parents had said, "Babies grow inside their mothers in a special place called the uterus."

Sexuality education is an ongoing process. Some parents may wish that a one-time lecture would suffice. But children's sexuality education starts long before that one-time talk and continues long after—through the media, advertising, the culture, interactions with friends and family members, sex education classes at school, and more. If you want to be your teen's main source of sexuality information, which also allows you to communicate your values, beliefs, and expectations, it's going to take more than a single sit-down.

Parents can be their children's first, best, and most important teachers about sexuality. How? By dealing with issues involving sexuality as they arise, whenever they arise, starting when their children are very young—and by answering questions openly and honestly at a level each child can understand.

When our daughter Jill was three years old, we conceived our second child. One evening when Amy was about seven months pregnant, she came home from a long day at the hospital, where she had been a Lamaze labor coach for another woman who delivered her baby that day. Amy arrived home just as Jill was getting ready for bed. That was always the most wonderful time in the evening, when we would all lie down together and cuddle.

On this night, Jill wasn't sleepy. Instead, she had a zillion questions.

"Is the new baby a boy or a girl?"

"A little boy," Amy said.

"Does it hurt when the baby comes out?"

"Sometimes, but that's why I was there as a labor coach—to help the mother do certain exercises so it wouldn't hurt."

"Will you coach me when I grow up and have a baby?"

"Absolutely, if that's what you want."

Amy hadn't slept for more than 24 hours. She was curled drowsily around Jill's body when Jill said, "Mommy, I have one more question."

Now, the one piece of information lacking in Jill's sexuality education at that point was how the daddy planted the seed. She knew that babies grow in the mother's uterus. She knew they come out through the vagina. But she didn't know about intercourse.

Amy thought, *Oh, no. Here it comes. Here I am, the sex educator, committed to honesty—and pregnant and exhausted. Do I really want to explain intercourse to a three-year-old? Is she ready for this?* Amy took a deep breath. Then she said, "What's your question, Toots?"

"Mommy," Jill said, "when we go to New York, are we taking the train or the car?"

What Jill was saying, in her childish way, was, "Okay, enough about babies. What about New York?"

Whether you're talking about sexuality with young children or teens, listen closely enough to hear what they're really asking. Keep the flow of information at their level. They'll let you know when they've heard enough to satisfy their curiosity. Leave the door to conversation open. When they want more, they'll come back.

Try to tailor your sexuality education program to the needs of your child. Some teens may respond to talking. Others would prefer to watch videos or go to the library to read books. Don't force your teen to read a particular book; just make it available. Having sexual information around the house and out in the open sends the message that it's okay to have sexual thoughts and feelings and to be curious. It lets your children know that sex is not a topic they have to sneak around or feel ashamed about. It also gives you some control over the sources they turn to for information.

JUST THE FACTS

In a national survey of teens and parents, 43 percent of the parents said that sex is a frequent topic of conversation in their homes. But only 26 percent of the teens said that their parents speak to them about sex with any regularity.[1]

What to Say When: A Sexuality Education Timeline

While every child is unique, certain types of sexual information are considered appropriate for certain developmental stages. This section gives you a general overview of what children can be taught at the various stages. Teens are last on the list, but you'll find the other descriptions useful if you have younger children. Specific information about many of these topics is found in "Part II: Issues to Know About and Talk About."*

EARLY CHILDHOOD

Use proper names for body parts. Girls and women have a vulva, clitoris, vagina, uterus, and ovaries. Boys and men have a penis, scrotum, and testicles. Read aloud age-appropriate sexually informative books. Talk about good touch and bad touch. Discuss the concept of privacy and present your values on masturbation. Be prepared for sexual exploration games. Help your child build respect and appreciation for her body. Help instill initiative, confidence, and respect for self and others.

MIDDLE CHILDHOOD (AGES 5–8): EARLY ELEMENTARY SCHOOL YEARS

Be open for questions that are best answered simply, factually, and concretely. Listen carefully and answer questions directly. Use opportunities to talk about sexuality and relationship issues as they arise (pets, TV, movies, books, the Internet, news). Reinforce self-respect and respect for others as well as positive decision making and assertive behavior.

PREADOLESCENCE (AGES 9–12): LATER ELEMENTARY SCHOOL YEARS

Give general information on how bodies will change for both sexes. Many children have not yet reached puberty but are curious about the facts. Give

---

* See also "Step 3: Understand Your Teen's Sexual Development" (pages 33–40).

them direct, concrete information and explain your value system. Make sure to include information about breast development, erections, menstruation, acne, ejaculation, wet dreams, masturbation, homosexuality, bisexuality, and reproduction. Continue to build self-respect and respect for others. Reinforce assertiveness and good decision making.

EARLY ADOLESCENCE (AGES 12–15): MIDDLE SCHOOL/JUNIOR HIGH SCHOOL YEARS

Provide more detailed information on body changes and puberty. Present topics like orgasm, pregnancy, birth control, sexually transmitted infections (STIs), the differences between what love is and isn't,* self-respect, assertiveness, alcohol and drug awareness, the importance of delaying intercourse, and alternatives to intercourse. Share your views on dating patterns. Talk about personal safety. Continue to reinforce your values.

ADOLESCENCE (AGES 15–18): HIGH SCHOOL YEARS

Provide information on safer sex practices. Continue to discuss assertiveness, peer pressure, and alcohol and drugs. Talk about abstinence, reasons to delay sexual intercourse, and alternative sexual behaviors. Reinforce information on STIs and birth control. More discussions on sexual orientation and on the differences between what love is and isn't may be helpful. Discuss ways to avoid sexual trauma (rape, abuse, harassment) and what to do if it does occur. Explain your values and why you hold them. Share your ideas on how to deal with people who hold different beliefs. Gradually allow for more independence, and reinforce responsible behavior.

JUST the FACTS

As teens get older and are more likely to be sexually active, their parents talk to them less about sex. In one national survey, 22 percent of twelve-year-olds reported that their parents "rarely/never" speak to them about sex. Among fifteen-year-olds, this figure rose to 58 percent.[2]

Building Communication Skills

Your teen wants your attention, recognition, acceptance, approval, love, and respect. If he knows he has these, he's more likely to take your guidance. But

---

* See "Is It Love?" on pages 50–51.

you can't just assume that he knows how you feel about him. You have to tell him—not only in words, but also in your actions and your general attitude.

High on the list of skills you need to communicate effectively with your teen is the ability to listen. Stand or sit in a relaxed, nonthreatening position. Avoid crossing your arms over your chest or placing your hands on your hips. Keep your facial expression open and inviting. Maintain eye contact (without staring or glaring) to show you're paying attention.

Listen without interrupting, except to summarize what your teen is saying. You might say, "I understand that this concert is important to you, and that all of your friends are going." This lets him know that you're paying attention.

What if you don't agree with what he's saying? Hear him out anyway. Wait your turn to talk. Remember that this is a discussion, not an opportunity for you to lecture. When you were a teen, did preaching, moralizing, criticizing, or nagging work with you? They're not going to work with your teen, either.

If your teen interrupts you while you're talking, you might say, "Please let me finish talking. I listened to you without interrupting. I'd appreciate it if you showed me the same consideration and respect."

In all of your discussions with your teen, try to communicate your faith in him as a growing young adult. Stay positive. Watch for opportunities to catch him showing good judgment, then affirm his behavior. When you disagree, don't automatically conclude that you're right and he's wrong. Maybe his position has merit. Think about it, then support him if it does. For example, if your family is going out to dinner and your teen suggests a new restaurant, go there if you can. Reinforce his ability to make good choices by saying things like, "You had a great idea. Thanks for sharing it."

HOW YOU SAY WHAT YOU SAY

Imagine that a parent and child are walking hand-in-hand along a quiet street. Suddenly, a big dog trots around the corner. The parent stiffens, grips the child's fingers tightly, and stammers, "D-d-don't be afraid of the d-d-dog."

What has the parent said to the child? Not to be afraid. What has the parent communicated to the child by the way she said it? To be very afraid. How is the child likely to feel? Confused.

A similar state of confusion can result during conversations about love, relationships, and sex. If we tell a teen that masturbation is perfectly normal and nothing to be embarrassed about, but we can't look him in the eye when we say it, our style undermines our message.

What we don't say can also send mixed messages. If we warn a young woman that men will lose respect for her if she has sex with them, but we don't tell her anything about her sexual choices, pleasure, or rights, we may give her a warped sense of her sexuality. If we talk openly with our teens about sex but never mention homosexuality, our silence on this topic may signal our disapproval.

When counseling adults, we often find that their sexual attitudes were shaped as much by what they weren't taught as by what they were. Many women in our practice were given the "nice-girls-don't" message when they were younger. When they finally married, they still viewed sex as something they shouldn't be interested in. We've also seen men who were told that sex should only be used as an expression of love. They were brought into therapy by their partners, who wanted to enjoy a broader range of sexual expression, like fun-sex or sex-sex.*

Sound decisions are based on a clear understanding of the issues. As you talk with your teen, stay alert to how you're saying what you're saying. Do your words match your body language? Your facial expression? Your tone of voice?

INTENT, MESSAGE, AND IMPACT

Not long ago, a family came into our office. The daughter flopped into a chair and wouldn't make eye contact. The father sat down, sighed with exasperation, and said, "I give up! I just can't get through to her!" The mother stayed silent. You could have cut the tension with a knife.

The father described the scene at the previous night's dinner table. Wanting to engage his daughter in conversation, he had asked, "What's on your calendar for the rest of the week?" In an agitated voice, she said, "Nothing!" He said, "What do you mean, nothing?" She replied, "What part of nothing don't you understand?" He persisted with, "Don't you have soccer practice?" She shouted, "My schedule's on the refrigerator! Do I have to read it to you?" Then she jumped up, left the table, and spent the rest of the evening in her room with the door closed. The father had no idea why his daughter had acted that way.

Communication can be broken down into three parts: the *intent*, the *message*, and the *impact*. The intent is the goal behind what the speaker is saying; it's what you want to accomplish with your message. The father's main intent was to engage his daughter in conversation about things that were important to her. His secondary intent may have been to show her that he was interested in her and her activities.

The second part of a communication is the message itself—the actual words. There doesn't seem to be anything wrong with, "What's on your calendar for the rest of the week?" But we know from the daughter's reaction that something wasn't right.

This brings us to the third part of communication—the impact, or how the message feels to the person on the receiving end. In effective communication, the message you send has the impact you intend. Clearly, that was

---

* For more on this topic, see "Love-Sex, Fun-Sex, and Sex-Sex" on pages 16–17.

not the case here. Fortunately, we were able to get the daughter to tell the story from her point of view.

Three weeks earlier, she explained, her father had insisted that everyone in the family write their schedules on the monthly calendar he had hung on the refrigerator. After some gentle coaxing, she said she had been "mortified" that now "everyone in the universe" would know that she had no social life. When her father had innocently asked about her schedule, the wound had been reopened. The father said he had no idea of the impact his question would have. He couldn't imagine that she felt the way she did.

He apologized for having hurt her feelings. The family agreed that from that point on, the calendar would be kept in a closed kitchen drawer. Then they began to deal with the real issue: how the daughter felt about her social life.

METACOMMUNICATION

When the impact of what you say doesn't match your intent, try *metacommunication*. This is a fancy word that simply means "communicating about the communication." You and the other person stop talking about *what* you were talking about and start exploring *how* you were talking.

When the father started noticing a problem in his conversation with his daughter (such as her attitude, tone of voice, and/or inappropriate energy level), he could have stopped what he was saying and focused on the process. He might have said, "Time out. We seem to be getting into hot water. Let's figure out what's going on." Or "Wait a minute. Please help me understand why you're upset."

GETTING BEHIND ANGER

Suppose your teen just left for a party she said was being chaperoned by her friend's parents. You go out to dinner, and as you walk into the restaurant, you spot those same parents sitting at another table. What's your first response? Anger.

Actually, your first response probably isn't anger. Anger is generally a secondary feeling—the result of other emotions like frustration, powerlessness, being hurt, and feeling betrayed.

Think of a recent time when you felt angry. Go behind the anger and ask yourself, "What was I frustrated about? Hurt by? What was making me feel powerless? Betrayed?"

When you get angry with your teen, take a mental step backward. Try to figure out what's behind your anger. This will stop you from responding in anger—shouting, frowning, wagging your finger, and saying things you might later regret. What do you do when someone approaches you in anger? You retreat or protect yourself by going on the offensive. So will your teen.

In his seminars, psychologist and author David Schnarch encourages people to speak from the best in themselves to the best in others.[3] When you speak from your anger, you belittle and demean your teen. You scare him away. When you speak from your hurt or frustration, you're more likely to speak from your softer side—the best in you at that time. And you're more likely to be heard.

Often, in the heat of anger, we use "You-statements." We start each sentence with "you." As in: "You lied to me." "You shouldn't have done that." "You can't be trusted." You-statements can be judgmental and accusatory. They can include name-calling, put-downs, and even threats. They don't speak from the best in you or to the best in your teen.

Try "I-statements" instead. Like: "I'm really hurt that you didn't tell me the truth." "I feel betrayed because you broke my trust." "I'm frustrated because we had an agreement—no parents, no parties—and you didn't keep your part of it." I-statements are a way to focus on your feelings instead of lashing out at your teen.

HANDLING DISAGREEMENTS

One of the jobs of being a teen is to challenge authority. Teens test limits. They argue. They disagree with their parents. They push. If you push back, you're in for a wearying battle of wills. The more you assert your authority, the more you affirm your teen's power in a negative way. If your teen could put this into words, he might say, "Look at how powerful I am. See how much power they have to use to subdue me."

It takes two people to have a power struggle. Be an Adult and sidestep gracefully.* Sidestepping the struggle doesn't mean sidestepping the issue. You can disagree in ways that don't discount your teen's point of view. Here are some examples:

- "I hear what you're saying, but I don't agree."
- "Let's agree to disagree. We don't have to agree on everything."
- "I'm sorry you feel that way."
- "I respect your right to have an opinion, but I don't feel the same way you do."
- "Let's suppose that what you're saying is true. Where does that take us in our discussion?"

Statements like these let your teen know that you acknowledge his position, even though you may not share it. This helps to create an open environment—one in which he'll feel more comfortable asking all kinds of questions, including sexual questions. It makes him an equal partner in the discussion. To develop the self-respect necessary to mature into a responsible Adult, a teen needs to feel appreciated as an individual. He needs to be

---

* See "The Miron Model" on pages 19–27.

recognized as a young adult with opinions worth hearing, not as a kid who has no voice.

Listen to your teen. Share your views on various subjects, explain why you feel as you do, but always be willing to listen. Over time, you and your teen will differ about many things. That's to be expected. How you disagree may be more important than what you disagree about.

FIGHTING FAIRLY

There's a myth that happy families don't fight. Many parents feel that when the family fights, something must be wrong. In fact, all families fight. Differing attitudes, values, experiences, likes, and dislikes—the things that make each member of your family wonderfully unique—will sometimes lead to conflict. When it happens, don't panic. And when someone tells you that her family never fights, don't believe her. She's not being truthful, she's in denial, or she's calling their fights something else—discussions, differences, misunderstandings.

What makes family life good or bad isn't whether conflict exists, but how people deal with it. Are your family fights mutually respectful? Do some people constantly have to get their way? Does one family member always have to win? Does anyone in your family tend to sulk, bully, use the silent treatment, lash out, or try to manipulate others during a fight?

Your whole family can fight fairly and constructively if you use a win-win model. This is something you may have to practice, since it probably won't come naturally. Our culture applauds competition. The model of conflict presented in competitive arenas like sports or business is a win-lose model. "May the best person win," we say. "To the victor belong the spoils." There's little respect for compromise, and a tie is not much better than a loss. In much of our world, either you win or you lose.

When you bring a win-lose model into a family (or any intimate relationship), problems result. For a family to work, all the members have to be on the same side. Either all of you win or you've all lost. If you walk away from a conflict with a family member and you feel like you've won, watch out. Chances are that person's Adolescent feels like a loser and can't wait to make you pay.

Effective conflict resolution requires a win-win model. When you and a family member disagree, take a step back and try to figure out what's most important. Is it getting your own way, or is it finding a solution that's acceptable to both of you? This doesn't mean that you should bury your feelings or automatically give up and give in. Be assertive—but be fair. Remember that the other person has feelings, too. Be open to the possibility of a compromise.

How can you know what the other person feels, wants, and needs? By listening. Don't just listen for a weak point in her argument—one you can exploit in order to promote your own agenda. Instead, listen with an open mind. If everyone in your family can learn this basic skill, everyone will benefit, and everyone will win.

Conversation Starters

Are certain topics off-limits in your home, or can family members talk about almost anything? The more open your home environment is, the more comfortable your teen will feel talking with you about sexual topics.

Just because your teen is asking questions about a sexual behavior doesn't mean he's engaged in it. On the other hand, if he isn't asking questions, you can't assume that he's not sexually active. As a parent, you can't wait for your teen to start a conversation. That's your responsibility.

Look for opportunities that allow an easy transition into discussions about sexual and relationship issues. These include the birth of a pet, song lyrics, a movie or television show, or the divorce of someone your teen knows. When the news reports that a married public official is being questioned about his relationship with a young intern, you might discuss sexual harassment, power differences in relationships, and your values on sexual loyalty and commitment. When a TV show makes fun of a group of people, such as gays or Jews or African Americans, wait for a commercial, then start a conversation about tolerating differences and how humor shouldn't hurt.

There are countless issues you can talk about with your teen. Here's a list of topics that may make interesting and informative conversation starters:

- What are the conditions that would make you feel ready for shared sexual activity?
- How do you feel about casual sex? Why do you feel that way?
- Do you think that birth control should be made available to minors?
- If you could only save a mother or her unborn child, which would you choose? Why?
- When does life begin? When sperm meets egg? When a fetus could survive outside the womb? At birth? What do you think?
- Are men and women different emotionally? If you think they are, how are they different?
- What do you think "masculine" means? What do you think "feminine" means? Can a woman be "masculine"? Can a man be "feminine"?
- Do you think that people choose their sexual orientation? Do they choose to be gay or straight? Do you think that gay people can be converted or convinced to be straight?
- What does it mean to be bisexual?
- What does it mean to be an adult?
- Do you think alcohol or drugs can influence someone's sexual decisions and behavior?

- Do you think it's possible for a single parent to raise a well-adjusted child?
- Do you think it's possible for a gay parent to raise a well-adjusted child?
- How involved should fathers be in raising children?
- What are some of the advantages and disadvantages of couples living together before marriage? Do you plan to wait until marriage? Why or why not?

Try This

Sit down with your teen and other family members you feel are appropriate for a discussion about controversial social or sexual issues. (These might include members of your extended family—grandparents, aunts and uncles, cousins.) Give everyone a sheet of paper and something to write with. Then give them instructions like the following, putting them in your own words.

1. *Divide the page into vertical columns—one for each person in our group, plus an extra column at the left.*

2. *In the far left column, list controversial social or sexual issues. Examples: abortion, birth control, same-sex marriage, masturbation, prostitution, legalizing drugs, premarital sex. (Invite everyone to contribute a topic.)*

3. *At the tops of the other columns, write the names of the other family members who are here with us.*

4. *Think about the issues. Think about the people in our group. Who would be in favor of each issue? Put a plus sign next to the issue in that person's column. Who would be against it? Put a minus sign next to the issue in that person's column.*

ISSUE	Mom	Dad	Simon	Terry	Aunt Barb
abortion	+	—	—	+	—
birth control	+	+	+	+	+
same-sex marriage	—	—	+	—	+

continued ⟶

Give people time to fill out their sheets. Afterward, share answers. How accurately were family members able to guess each other's beliefs? Discuss why you agree or disagree on an issue and why you thought others would feel a certain way.

Choosing Your Words

You're ready to start a discussion with your teen about a sexual topic. You know what your position is; you've thought long and hard about it. But every time you find a convenient opening, you freeze. What words should you use? What words shouldn't you use? What kind of language is right—and wrong?

Many parents ask themselves these questions. They want to talk with their teen, but they can't decide what to say. If you use technical words like fellatio or cunnilingus, will your teen understand what you're talking about? If you use slang, will she think you're trying to be cool—or will she laugh because the slang you use is hopelessly out of date? You might try what we do when we teach courses or workshops in sexuality. We start with the technical words, then introduce other common vocabulary, which includes slang and baby talk. Then we explain that in our course or workshop, we prefer the technical words. Slang changes, and often it's too crude for polite conversation.

You might tell your teen, "Fellatio is the correct and technical word for oral sex on a penis. You're probably going to hear lots of other terms for it, like 'blow job,' 'going down,' or 'giving head.' When we talk about fellatio, I'd prefer if we both called it by its real name." Or you might ask your teen which term she feels most comfortable using. If it's okay with you, you can both agree to use that instead. As an interesting side topic, you might point out how few tender and loving words we have for sexual behaviors—and explore some possible reasons why.

Whatever language you want your teen to use with you, try not to let your discomfort get in your way. Admit your discomfort and talk anyway. Isn't that what you want your teen to do?

HONESTY VS. CONFESSION

You've committed to being open and honest with your teen about sexual matters. Does that mean you must share the intimate details of your own sexual history and behavior? No. Confession should not be a part of sexuality education.

This is not being hypocritical. If your sexual values include the belief that your sexual behavior is a private matter—and most people's do—then questions about whether you had intercourse before marriage, for example, are out of bounds. You're under no obligation to answer them directly. Make it clear to your teen that this information is in a file marked "Personal & Confidential," and there it will remain. Make it equally clear that as a parent, you'll need to ask her some personal questions in order to help guide, educate, and protect her. Promise her that when she's an adult, you'll stop asking questions, because then her sex life will be private, too.

If your teen persists in asking personal questions, try to find out why. Is she putting you on the spot, or is she seeking information that might help her make a decision? If she's asking when you had sex for the first time, perhaps she's asking herself, "Am I ready to have sex now, or should I wait?"

You can respond to personal questions in a way that doesn't reveal your personal history. For example, if your teen asks, "Do you have oral sex?" you might respond, "Why do you want to know?" If she says, "I'm just curious," you can ask where her curiosity comes from. If she says, "I'm hearing a lot about it at school," you can talk about that. If it seems that she's considering whether oral sex is something she should be doing, you can ask her how this fits into (or doesn't fit into) her personal values. And if, in fact, she's just being nosy, you can tell her that what you do or don't do is right for you—and private.

POSITIVE VS. NEGATIVE MESSAGES

Many parents try to scare their teens away from behaviors they disapprove of, or they warn them away by saying, "Don't _____ [fill in the blank]." But fear-based approaches and don'ts don't work.

Some colleges put wrecked cars on campus before spring break to remind students to drive slowly and not to drink and drive. Students slow down to look at the cars, then speed up to find the best parking spaces. The impact of fear-based approaches is often short-lived. Rather than tell your teen what not to do, help him set goals he'll want to work toward—like a loving, long-term, respectful relationship with a committed partner. This, too, is part of sexuality education.

If you use fear and don'ts to teach, when your teen is ready for shared sexual expression, he'll have to undo any negative messages he has received in order to enjoy the experience. In our practice, we see many adults who still feel the effects of fear-based messages in their marriages.

Offer positive images of the joy of sharing sexual expression for the first time within the context you believe is right. You might tell your teen that everyone who has been sexually active, no matter how old they are now, can still remember their first time. Remind him that his first time will only happen once. Encourage him to choose the person, place, and time thoughtfully and carefully.

REINFORCEMENT, ENCOURAGEMENT, PUNISHMENT, AND LOGICAL CONSEQUENCES

What's the main goal of parenting a teen? To raise a responsible Adult. To accomplish this, you need to shift your focus from what you as a parent think to what your teen thinks. Instead of guiding the Child in your teen, you need to gradually shift that responsibility to your teen's Adolescent and emerging Adult.

Reinforcement and punishment are tools that can help you do this. Encouragement and the use of logical consequences are even more effective.

Behavior that leads to positive results—getting what you want and feeling good about it—tends to be repeated. Try to catch your teen behaving in ways you value, and reinforce those behaviors. For example, when your teen clears the table without being asked or reminded, don't just say, "Good job." Be more specific and say, "I'm delighted to see you clearing the table. Thanks. I really appreciate it." Whenever you can, notice times when your teen is using good judgment, following rules, and behaving responsibly. Then let her know how proud of her you are.

Focus on how your teen feels about herself, and encourage her positive feelings. Point out the sense of integrity she is building by behaving well, and comment on how that must feel. You might say, "I'll bet you feel good about . . ." or "Aren't you proud of yourself?" That's encouragement, and it goes a long way.

Reinforcing and encouraging positive behavior not only keeps the emotional environment pleasant between you and your teen. It also increases the chances that desired behaviors will be repeated. It's much more effective than punishment in pointing your teen in the right direction.

Punishment is often misunderstood. It may suppress or decrease the frequency of a behavior . . . for a while. It does not, however, eliminate or stop the behavior.

Imagine that you're speeding along the highway when you spot a state trooper in your rearview mirror. Almost without thinking, you ease up on the gas pedal. Your eyes go automatically to the speedometer, and you probably stay within a few miles of the posted speed limit—as long as the trooper is behind you. But as soon as the trooper pulls off the highway, what happens to your speed?

That's how punishment works. If the punishing agent or the threat of punishment is present, you get compliance. But as soon as the punishing agent or threat is gone, so is compliance. When a parent's only form of behavior management is punishment, a teen is more likely to spend time figuring out how to get around it than learning the appropriate behavior.

This is not to suggest that improper behavior shouldn't be punished. But punishment works best when used in tandem with reinforcement, logical consequences, and encouragement to behave appropriately.

Rather than policing your family, treat it as a team. As team members, children benefit when they do what's reasonably expected of them. When they don't, they lose some of the privileges of being on the team. That's a logical consequence.

Team members need to understand what's expected of them and what the consequences are for actions that don't meet expectations. Whenever possible, the penalties for misbehavior should be spelled out in advance. You might create a contract with your teen that goes something like this: "If you do this [an inappropriate behavior], then understand that this [a logical consequence] is going to happen. The choice will be yours." Always try to reinforce and encourage the positive option, and emphasize your faith in your teen's ability to make the right decision. Make it clear that your teen isn't losing a privilege forever, just for a certain period of time or until certain requirements are met. Leave a window of opportunity open for your teen to show his better side.

One of the privileges of being on a team is having a voice in family matters. Show respect for your teen by listening to his opinions about consequences he feels are too harsh. Consider whether the punishment fits the crime and whether it's practical. You and your teen don't have to agree, but try to work out your differences cooperatively. Inappropriate punishments send the message that you're trying to control his life instead of guiding him toward responsible self-control.

Often, as your teen tests his limits, your patience will get stretched. In the heat of the moment, it's tempting to make extravagant threats you can't enforce. For example, let's say you have a rule that no friends are allowed in the house unless an adult is present. You learn that your son has broken the rule by having his girlfriend over when you were away. You might announce, "I'm NEVER going to let you stay alone in the house again!" That may reflect your feelings at the moment, but it's not realistic.

It's far more constructive to find a logical consequence. For example, you might tell your teen, "Because you broke our rule, I can't trust you to stay at home alone for a while. For the next month, whenever I go out, you'll either have a sitter or go to your grandmother's house. When the month is up, I'll give you the chance to stay alone again and earn my trust. If you break the rule again, the punishment will double to two months." Stay calm and avoid speaking in a hostile or angry voice.

Always try to make the teen responsible for the outcome. Your role is to provide logical consequences for your teen's poor choices. Ultimately, he's responsible for his own actions—and the results of those actions.

When your teen is in error, speak to the best in him from the best in you. It's probably easier to do this with a three-year-old who disobeys than with an older teen who (you think and hope) should know better. Try to remember that inside that exasperating, confrontational teen is the same Child who has always needed your love, support, and encouragement. Expecting the best encourages the best in him.

> ## Try This
>
> In "Step 1: Define Your Goals and Values," a "Try This" exercise asked you to list the goals you have for your teen as a fully sexually educated young adult.* Look back at your list. With your goals in mind, what rules, contracts, and consequences have you established with your teen? Have you made your expectations clear? What will happen if your teen breaks a rule or ignores a contract? Does your teen know what will happen? If you haven't yet decided on or communicated your rules, contracts, and consequences, you may want to call a family meeting for this purpose. Prevention is your best form of management.

What If Your Teen Won't Talk with You?

If your teen never wants to discuss sexual issues, address that directly. You may want to explain that it's okay to feel uncomfortable, but there are some things she needs to do even if they are uncomfortable, and discussing sexual issues may be one of them.

Ask your teen why she's avoiding the subject, then listen and problem solve. You might say, "You seem to be quiet when it comes to questions about sexuality. If you had a question or concern, would you come to me?" Then follow up with conversation based on what you hear. Or say, "I'm concerned that you don't seem interested in talking with me about any sexuality issues. Why? Is there something I'm doing or not doing that's creating a problem?"

If your teen admits that it's hard to talk about sex with you because you're her parent, try saying, "I'm sorry you feel that way, but I can't help being your parent. Why don't you give me a couple of chances and see how we do?"

If your teen still resists conversation with you, you might recommend that she talk with someone else. This should be a person you trust who shares or is willing to voice your values, and also someone your teen likes and respects. You might tell your teen, "Even though I wish you'd talk with me about sex, if it's really too uncomfortable for you, why not talk with [name of person]?" Of course, you'll want to clear this with the other person first.

---

* Find this exercise on pages 12–13.

Letting Go

Teens, like adults, want a life that's purposeful and meaningful. You can help your teen achieve that goal. Let him know that you're aware of his growing need for independence, and give him many opportunities to make his own decisions.

Help your teen develop self-respect and self-reliance by showing respect for him. Involve him in family decision making whenever possible. Solicit his opinions when you can. Help him feel empowered and important. Recognize his voice, and give him a choice of options that are acceptable to you.

Gradually transfer more responsibility to your teen. If you give him a clothing allowance, make it clear that when the money's spent, you're not going to supplement it—and then don't. You may want to set some ground rules concerning inappropriate clothing, but be sure to communicate your confidence in his ability to make good decisions.

Give credit where credit is due. Notice and acknowledge your teen's behaviors, small and large, that make family life go smoothly. Avoid comparing him to his siblings or other teens. Emphasize the unique gifts that he brings to your family—the traits and talents that set him apart and make him special.

Show an interest in his life. Take the time to ask how he's doing and learn what's going on with him. Keep current with his interests—as current as you can, since they may change frequently.

You and your teen are writing your family's history. Today's page is blank. Write something you'll be proud to read twenty years from now.

BE PREPARED FOR ALMOST ANYTHING

Remember when your child was an infant and you traveled everywhere with diapers, a change of clothes, extra baby food, towels, toys—everything you might conceivably need? Chances are you never used half that stuff, but parents learn early on that it's best to be prepared.

It's the same now that your child is older. If you think through your position on various sexuality and relationship issues, you'll be equipped to deal with almost anything.

In this step, you'll consider some of the issues that may come up with your teen. They also may not come up, but thinking on your feet is easier if you know where you stand in the first place.

Privacy

At some point in their lives, many kids hang signs on their doors saying something like, "Keatia's Room: No Trespassing." The demand for emotional and physical privacy isn't aimed only at brothers and sisters. Parents need to respect a teen's privacy as well.

If you want to earn your teen's trust, respect for her privacy is a giant step in the right direction. Let her know that it's okay to keep some thoughts and feelings private, but you're always there for her if she wants to talk. When she does share something with you, reinforce how much it means to you and how much you appreciate it. If she feels the need to hold back, respect that, too. If her reticence hurts you, tell her.

No matter how curious you are about what she's up to, sneaking through the contents of drawers or glove compartments—or reading journals, diaries, or private correspondence (including email)—is almost always out of line. When is it not? If you believe your teen is suicidal or in danger, or you suspect she's using drugs or making a pipe bomb—in other words, only in the most extreme situations. Your teen can see through excuses like, "I was trying to find your red T-shirt so I could wash it, and I accidentally saw something you wrote in your diary." What you're really saying (and what she hears) is, "I don't trust you, so I've been snooping through your things."

If you have a reason to be worried about your teen, say so. For example, what if her best friend's mom calls to say that she found birth control pills in her daughter's underwear drawer? You might tell your teen, "Jen's mom found birth control pills in her drawer. I'm worried. Do you have any surprises for me?" Follow up with something like, "I hope you'll come and talk with me directly if you're thinking about the need for birth control. I'm here for you." Talk about your concerns. Don't compromise your integrity by spying.

Keep your private life private, too. If you have books or videos on sexuality that are not appropriate for your children to see, keep them hidden and out of reach. Make it clear that the right to privacy goes both ways. You won't tolerate her looking through Mom's purse or Dad's wallet or prying open a locked chest in the basement storage room.

If you find your teen digging through your closet, or you realize that your private things have been disturbed, be direct. You might say something like, "Those are my private things, and they're meant for me alone. I don't appreciate you going through them any more than you'd like me going through your things." You might ask what she was looking for and why.

We know one parent who found his daughter rummaging through his nightstand drawer. When he questioned her, she said, "I thought I might find a condom. I was curious about what they look like." This gave him the opportunity to talk with her about respect for privacy, as well as the importance of coming to him directly with a question. Once their family privacy boundaries were back in place, he showed her a condom and explained how and when to use one.

When You Walk In on Your Teen

You thought your son was downstairs, busy on the computer. Carrying an armload of clean laundry, you kick open his bedroom door and—oops!—he's masturbating.

The first thing you need to do is apologize for invading his privacy. Then leave. Later, you can talk about what happened. If you accept masturbation as a safe, healthy form of self-expression, you might say, "I'm sorry I walked in on you. It was embarrassing for both of us. Masturbation is natural and nothing to feel bad about, but it's private. I apologize for barging into your room. I won't do it again."

If you believe that masturbation is wrong, let your emotions settle before talking with your teen. Then apologize for walking in on him, explain your position on masturbation, and give your reasons for feeling as you do.

Imagine another scenario. You come home from the movies to find your son and his girlfriend naked and entwined on the couch. Your first impulse may be to react in anger. That's understandable, but it's not productive.

Instead, take a deep breath. Try to figure out what's behind your anger. Are you shocked and disappointed to learn that he's sexually active when you don't want him to be? Has he lied to you about being sexually active? Has he broken a rule about having friends in the house when you're not there? You'll need to address each issue separately.

Don't embarrass your teen in front of his girlfriend. Ask them both to please get dressed, then leave the room. Return in a few moments and say that it's time for the girlfriend to go home. If she can get there on her own, that's fine. If your son needs to take her home, allow him to do that. If she needs other transportation, suggest that she call her parents, or drive her home yourself. Stay calm and don't lecture. It won't be comfortable for either of you, but that's to be expected.

Then take some time to cool off and put your Adult in charge before you approach your teen.* Start with a positive statement—something like, "I love you, and you're very important to me." Then express your disappointment and your hurt. You might say, "I'm really disturbed [or troubled by, or upset about] what just happened," or "This is not the kind of behavior I expect or will tolerate," or "It's hard for me to trust you when you break rules."

If you walked in on sexual behaviors that you've asked your teen to abstain from or postpone, you could say, "If I can't trust you, I can't leave you at home unsupervised." You may be tempted to punish him or threaten punishment. Be careful. Under the circumstances, it's easy to say something you don't mean and can't possibly enforce.

It's common for parents who find their teens in compromising positions to blame the other teen. "My son would never have done that if his girlfriend hadn't seduced him." "My daughter would never have given in if she hadn't been pressured." This feeds the "you-and-me-against-the-world" feeling that is already a powerful part of many teen relationships. Try to separate the deed from the doer. Focus on the behavior. Explain why you find it unacceptable, then make it clear that you won't tolerate it.

What if your teen insists that he's in love? Don't dismiss his feelings, and avoid saying things like, "You only *think* you're in love. You have no idea what love really means." Instead, acknowledge his feelings. Then explain that love is not a good enough reason to break a promise, compromise your trust, and engage in risky behavior. Explain why you feel he's too young to support the consequences of sexual activity. Let him know that there are many ways to express love. Suggest that he and his girlfriend can hold hands, cuddle, take long walks together, talk on the phone, share their dreams, and engage in other behaviors you consider appropriate for his age and situation. Be specific about which behaviors you consider out of bounds.

---

* See "The Miron Model" on pages 19–27.

If you discover or suspect that your teen is sexually active, it's critical that you talk with him immediately about safer sex practices, condom use, sexually transmitted infections (STIs), and birth control, if you haven't already done so.* If it has happened once, it may happen again, even if you ask your teen to refrain.

When you give him this information, you're not giving him permission to be sexual. You can make that clear by saying something like, "You know how strongly I believe that teens your age should not engage in sexual intercourse. You know that I think it's wrong. But as your parent, I'm responsible for giving you information about safer sex now so you'll have it later in life. It's kind of like learning the rules of the road when you're fourteen. You can learn how to drive a car safely, but you can't and shouldn't drive. By giving you information about safer sex, I'm not saying that it's okay for you to have sex."

When Your Teen Walks In on You

What if your teen accidentally walks in on you when you're engaging in sexual activity? Stay calm. Address your mutual embarrassment, but don't make a big deal out of it.

Parents sometimes fear that a child will be traumatized by seeing them engaging in sexual activity. Our experience as sex therapists suggests that if the situation is handled constructively, it doesn't have to be traumatic for the child.

There's no magic formula for dealing with the situation. How you handle it will depend on the age of the child, what she observed, how much she knows about sexual behavior, and how upset or confused she is. While an older teen may only need a reminder of the necessity to respect other people's privacy, a younger child may require an explanation of what she saw. Keep your explanation as simple as possible and at a level appropriate for the child's age.

The old adage "An ounce of prevention is worth a pound of cure" fits here. Protect your privacy by locking your bedroom door before you engage in sexual activity. Explain people's need for privacy early in your children's lives, and make it a family policy that a closed door is to be respected. Remember to extend the same courtesy to your teen.

When Your Teen Lies to You

In an attempt to get away with something, or to at least minimize the consequences, people will sometimes lie, and teens are no exception. For example, suppose that your daughter has a friend over when you're out for the evening. You know she did, because a neighbor saw the friend arrive and

---

* See "Issue 5: Safer Sex" (pages 170–205).

told you. But when you ask your daughter, "Was [name of the friend] here?" she says, "No."

Try to impress on your teen the tremendous harm a lie can do. Not only does it create immediate problems, but it also makes you wonder whether she's lied in the past. Lies undermine trust; trust is hard to earn and even more difficult to reestablish once lost. If your teen has lied, you might say, "I'm really hurt that you lied to me. Lying undermines my trust in you, and it undermines your integrity in your own eyes. Is what you did really worth all that?" It may be that the lie is worse than your teen's misbehavior. If so, you can mention that as well.

What about consequences? We've borrowed an idea from a common road sign: "Work Zone: Speeding Fines Doubled." We suggest that if the teen disobeys but tells the truth, the normal consequences hold. If she disobeys and lies about it, the penalty doubles.

What if she doesn't tell an outright lie, but instead stretches or evades the truth? For example, when you ask, "Was [name of the friend] here?" she says, "No one was here this evening." Maybe your teen defines "evening" as the time of the day between 6:00 P.M. and 9:00 P.M., and her friend didn't arrive until "night"—after 9:00 P.M. Make it clear that a lie is a lie, and the results are the same.

Teen Pregnancy

Your daughter has something to tell you. You wonder what it could be. Did she get an A on that science test she studied so hard for? Was she elected to represent her church youth group? You eagerly anticipate her announcement. She looks at you and says, "I think I'm pregnant."

Or your son, who's just been accepted to college on a basketball scholarship, announces that he's going to get a job instead. Why? Because his girlfriend is pregnant with his child.

You've always told yourself, "That can't happen to my daughter/son." What do you do if it does?

Your first priority is to support your child. No matter how angry, frustrated, or disappointed you may feel, saying, "How could you?" or "I warned you about this!" is not constructive. Avoid accusations, and be careful not to blame the teen's partner. Be open to your teen's feelings, fears, and anxieties, and share your own concerns. Problem solve collectively, but pour on the love and support. A life crisis can pull a family apart, or it can provide the opportunity to cement bonds.

Your second priority is to learn if the teen really is pregnant. Is she panicking because her period is a little late? Has she taken a home pregnancy test? Has a doctor or clinic confirmed the pregnancy? Is emergency contraception still a possibility?

THE SIGNS OF PREGNANCY

The signs of pregnancy include:

- a missed period
- nausea/vomiting
- inexplicable fatigue
- sore or enlarged breasts
- headaches
- frequent urination

BUT . . .

- For many women, especially young women, irregular periods (missed periods or changes in the menstrual cycle) are normal. They can happen from month to month. They may be caused by worry, stress, illness, travel, excessive exercise, or excessive weight gain or loss.
- Nausea and vomiting may be caused by food poisoning, stress, and other stomach disorders.
- Fatigue can be caused by stress, depression, the common cold or flu, or getting too little sleep.
- Sore or enlarged breasts may be a sign that menstruation is about to begin.
- Headaches may be caused by stress, caffeine withdrawal, eye strain, and any number of other factors.
- Frequent urination may be caused by a urinary tract infection, diabetes, or taking diuretics. Some teens take diuretics for weight loss.

SO . . .

A pregnancy test done by a medical professional is the surest way to find out if your teen is really pregnant.

Home pregnancy tests rarely show a false positive, but it's not unusual to get a false negative. If a woman takes a home pregnancy test and it says she is not pregnant, she should take the test again after another week. If she hasn't had another act of unprotected intercourse, the second test should be pretty accurate. Planned Parenthood, local women's health centers, and church-supported pregnancy centers will not only test for pregnancy but will also provide counseling about the options available.

If your daughter is pregnant, there are many issues to consider. Should she keep the baby? If not, would she consider emergency contraception or abortion, or is that against her principles? What's the baby's father's position on abortion? What's involved in putting a baby up for adoption? If she chooses to keep the baby, how will she support herself and the child? Will the baby's father be involved in financial support and/or childrearing? Are you, as a parent, willing or able to assist with raising the baby? What about the father's family?

If your teen is the father, encourage him to be an active participant in the decisions about the pregnancy and to support his partner emotionally and financially. He (and you) should not put all the responsibility on the young woman. For example, if abortion is the best option, he can help pay for it and be there to provide emotional support.

How you handle this pregnancy will be crucial to your child's well-being later in life, and to your relationship with your child. You and your teen are going to have to live with your decisions forever. As a parent, you may want to push your own agenda. Your instinctive urge to protect your child will be very strong. Don't try to talk or bully your teen into doing what you think should be done.

Do let your teen know your position on the various issues. Either you'll help raise the child, or you won't be able to. Either you don't believe in abortion, or you think abortion is the most practical option under the circumstances. Either you support adoption, or you oppose it. Meanwhile, listen to your teen's thoughts, feelings, and positions. Make it clear that you'll keep loving your child no matter what.

JUST THE FACTS

■ In the United States, there are nearly one million teen pregnancies each year and about half as many teen births. The U.S. has the highest rates of teen pregnancy and birth by far of any comparable country.[1]

■ The vast majority (78 percent) of pregnancies among teens are not fully planned or intended.[2]

■ Compared to women who delay childbearing, teen mothers are less likely to complete high school and more likely to end up on welfare.[3]

Body Art and Body Piercing

Your teen may be dying to get a tattoo or have her tongue pierced. Many teens believe that tattoos are sexy, and that piercings enhance oral sex. When you object, she might say, "What's the big deal? Everyone's doing it," or "I'll get the tattoo where no one will even see it."

You may have many reasons to want to talk your teen out of her decision. To begin with, explain the health concerns. Dirty tattoo instruments can introduce a host of infections including the human immunodeficiency virus (HIV, the cause of AIDS). Tongue studs can crack teeth. Navel piercings can get infected when clothing rubs against them. Genital piercing complications can cause difficulties with sexual response. All piercings have potential problems.

But it may not be just the health issues that concern you. You may not like the message that tattoos and piercings send—and years down the road, your teen might not either. Remind your teen that tattoos and the scars from piercings are permanent. She may think it's the greatest thing now, but ask her to consider how she'll feel about it when she's 20 or 40 or 60. Some tattoos are potent symbols. Will she still want to be wearing that symbol in a year or two or ten from now?

If you decide to support your teen's decision, check out the person and place where she's going to do it. Have her contact your local Health Department and Better Business Bureau office to learn if any complaints have been filed. Encourage her to talk with people who have had it done and find out what the downside is; there almost always is a downside. As with all decisions, sexual and otherwise, solid information is your best ally.

Pornography

The marvels of the Internet are astounding. You can communicate freely with people from around the world. You can play bridge with three people from Kalamazoo, buy and sell common or rare objects, and learn all about that drug your sister's doctor just prescribed for her. Your teen can do research for a school project from your home computer.

But there's no such thing as a one-sided coin. Although the Internet is wonderful in many ways, it's full of dangers as well, and they're not limited to computer viruses. If you have Internet access, chances are that your teen has been (or soon will be) exposed to pornography of all types.

What is pornography? The definition varies from person to person and from community to community. However, a basic definition would be material that is explicit and is designed to arouse. Many parents believe pornography is inappropriate for their teen (and maybe for themselves and their partners, too, depending on their personal or religious values). This may be particularly true for pornography that depicts sex without affection, commitment, respect, or consequences.

Protecting your teen isn't easy, but there are things you can do. You can ask directly if he has seen pornography on the Internet, or you can ask hypothetically, "What would you do if you were surfing the Web and you stumbled across a pornographic site?" Share your thoughts and feelings about pornography, and explain why you believe as you do. Ask how he feels about it.

You might point out that what he sees at a pornographic site is only one type of sexual expression.* If it's the only type he sees, he might get a skewed vision of sexual behavior and an unrealistic idea of responsible relationships, body types, and intimate activities. If you're uncomfortable talking with him about pornography, explain why, if you can. Try not to let your discomfort stop you from protecting your teen.

There are ways to minimize your teen's opportunities to explore pornographic sites. Placing your computer in an open area or limiting the number of hours he spends on the computer (especially unsupervised) might help. You can also block certain sites on the Internet (and the adult channels on cable TV, if you have it). Ask your service provider what controls are available. You can buy parental controls at computer stores or download them from various Internet sites.

Even if you take these preventive steps, don't get too comfortable. Someone else's parents might not be as vigilant as you. And pornography is available in many other forms—magazines, DVDs, movies, videos. You can't block them all. That's why it's important to inoculate your teen with your values as well as with information.

Sexual Predators

You want your teen to feel confident about herself and the world she lives in. You've taught her right from wrong, good from bad. You want her to be friendly and kind to others. But the world is a complex place, and there are people who will try to take advantage of your teen. They're called predators, and in the sexual arena their impact can be long-term and devastating.

What does a predator look like? Just like you or me. Predators come from all races, classes, religions, and professions, but they usually show a special interest in children or teens. If they don't organize their work or careers around children, they frequently volunteer in positions that will put them in contact with young people.

Does this mean that you should suspect everyone who has a special interest in kids? Is every teacher, coach, youth leader, counselor, mentor, and scout leader a potential or actual predator? Of course not. Most of the adults who devote themselves to the enrichment of young people's lives are caring, dedicated role models. Some aren't, and that's why you need to talk with your teen.

Talk about good touch and bad touch. You might say, "Affection is great, but it shouldn't make you uncomfortable. If someone is touching you in a way or place that you don't like, please tell me." Or "While most people you

---

* For more on this topic, see "Love-Sex, Fun-Sex, and Sex-Sex" on pages 16–17.

meet are safe, you need to keep your radar turned on. Some people take advantage of children and teens in many ways, including sexually."

Talk about how anonymous the Internet and chat rooms are. Explain that not everyone is honest, and that "Jennifer," the neat fifteen-year-old friend your teen met online, may actually be Jack, a forty-five-year-old pedophile. Stress that she should *never* give out personal information—her full name, telephone number, address, the school she attends, where she'll be on Friday night—under any circumstances. Make sure that she understands and agrees to this rule.

Talk about the fact that no one, under any circumstances, has the right to be sexually inappropriate with your teen. This includes people in positions of authority—teachers, coaches, religious leaders, doctors, mentors, youth leaders, family friends, friends' parents, and other adults. It includes uncles, aunts, cousins, stepparents, and older siblings. Let your teen know that she can come to you whenever she feels uncomfortable about anything. You might say, "If anyone ever touches you or approaches you in a way that makes you feel strange, uncomfortable, or afraid, I want you to tell me right away."

Explain that it's normal for young people to have crushes on older people, like a favorite teacher or an interesting friend of the family. What isn't normal, healthy, or appropriate is for an older person to return the attention in a romantic or sexual way. Say that if and when that happens, you want to know about it.

What if your teen tells you that an adult has behaved inappropriately? What if the adult is someone you know, maybe even your best friend? Your first impulse might be to say, "I'm sure he didn't mean anything by it." That may or may not be true, but it's not the first thing you should say. By even slightly defending the adult in question, you may be sending your teen the message that you're not taking her seriously. On the other hand, your first response probably shouldn't be to pick up the phone and call the police.

Instead, thank your teen for coming to you and talking with you. Tell her that's what you want her to do. Then get as much additional information from your teen as you can. Was this an isolated incident? If so, it may be open for misinterpretation. Or does there seem to be a pattern? Did the adult ask or instruct your teen to keep the incident a secret? Does your teen know anyone else who has had a similar experience with that person? Were there any witnesses? What exactly happened? What was said? What was done? Ask for specific details, but let your teen provide them. Don't put words in her mouth or thoughts in her head.

The information you receive will determine your next step. If the behavior in question is open for interpretation, you might want to go to the adult, explain your teen's discomfort, and request that he keep an appropriate distance from your teen. If the adult really is okay, that should be sufficient, and the situation won't happen again. If the behavior is not open for interpretation—if it's clear that the adult made a direct sexual advance to your teen—then you do need to report it to the police. Predators don't offend once. By taking action, not only are you protecting your teen. You may be protecting hundreds of other teens.

If your best friend keeps telling your son how handsome he is and it's making him uncomfortable, ask your friend to stop. You don't have to accuse your friend of child molestation. Simply tell her that her comments, however well-intentioned they may be, are having a negative impact on your son. You might say something like, "I'm sure you don't mean anything wrong by telling my son he's handsome. But it's making him feel uncomfortable. I'd appreciate your not saying that to him anymore."

Sexual Harassment

Your teen should know what sexual harassment is—and isn't. Explain that sexual harassment is sexually oriented behavior that is uninvited, unwelcome, and unwanted. It is not the same as flirting. Flirtation usually happens between two people who are playing the same game, and it's pleasurable to both parties. Harassment typically occurs when one person has more power than the other. That power can be formal, like the power a teacher has over a student, a boss over an employee, or a religious leader over a member of the congregation. It can be informal, like the power a popular kid has over others in a group, or the power a group has over an individual.

JUST THE FACTS

- According to one national survey, four out of five students have experienced some type of sexual harassment in school. This includes both girls and boys.[4]

- For many students, sexual harassment is an ongoing experience. More than one in four students report experiencing it often.[5]

- Nearly all students say they know what harassment is. Sixty-nine percent of students say their school has a policy on sexual harassment. But harassment is still widespread in America's schools.[6]

Your teen has the legal right to a school or work environment free of sexual harassment. Behavior with a real or implied sexual content can't be labeled harassment, however, if the offender doesn't know that the other person is offended. If your teen is bothered by something that is said or done at school, he needs to make that clear to the person who is bothering him. He should also inform adults in authority—a teacher, a coach, a school counselor, the principal, his employer.

Explain to your teen that unwanted sexual matter can include jokes about gays or lesbians, talk about sex at the lunch table, being touched or brushed against, or comments about his clothes or body. Once your teen warns the offender that he's not comfortable with the behavior, he should keep a journal of what is said and when. Have him write the offender's reactions as well. If other people heard the conversation, he should include their names. If the comments continue, it's sexual harassment, and he can pursue legal remedies.

PHYSICAL HARASSMENT

Most people agree that unwelcome and uninvited kissing and sexually explicit fondling are clear examples of sexual harassment. But some people, especially teens, are less clear about such things as touching, patting, pinching, stroking, or brushing up against someone. These actions make your teen uncomfortable, but the person isn't really doing anything wrong, is he? Suppose it's just accidental? Mentioning it could be embarrassing.

Tell your teen not to put up with it. A single instance of, for example, brushing against her body while she's walking the hallway or climbing into a car might be accidental (though she should certainly expect an apology). But repeated physical contact is not. Your teen should tell the offender that she finds such behavior offensive and she wants it to stop immediately. In most states, she can even seek legal remedies. No one has the right to touch her body without her permission.

WHAT TO DO?

Situation:
Your teen says he's quitting basketball. When you ask him about it, he says he's uncomfortable with how the assistant coach touches him.

Suggestions:
Ask him to talk with the assistant coach, clearly describing the behavior and how it made him feel. Another adult—you, the principal, the school counselor—should also be present during that conversation. Have your teen make a detailed account in writing of exactly what happened, when and where, who did and said what, how he felt, and the names of any witnesses. Find out if any of his teammates have had similar experiences. This kind of behavior is usually a pattern, not a one-time event. Reassure your teen that it isn't okay and shouldn't be tolerated. He shouldn't have to pay the price for someone else's problem.

NONPHYSICAL HARASSMENT

Not all sexual harassment involves actual contact. There are many forms of harassment that aren't physical. They include:

- unsolicited sexual propositions and sexual references
- unwanted phone calls of a sexual nature, whether the caller is a stranger or someone your teen knows
- wolf whistles, kissing sounds, and lewd remarks, often directed by groups of kids toward members of the other sex
- sexual slurs, dirty jokes, and innuendoes, if they persist in the presence of someone who has made it clear that they're unwelcome
- leering looks or a suggestive tone of voice that give sexual meanings to otherwise innocent remarks
- certain gestures

Regarding gestures, every culture has a sexual "sign language." But what's lewd in some cultures is entirely innocent in others. The American "okay" sign—making a ring with the thumb and forefinger—is obscene in some parts of Latin America. In some parts of the world, a man who looks full into the face of an unmarried woman is committing sexual harassment.

WHAT TO DO?

Situation:
Your son mentions that another student tells a lot of sexual jokes, and it makes him uncomfortable.

Suggestions:
Tell him to let the offender know how the jokes make him feel, and be clear that he wants them to stop. Ask him to keep a detailed written account of what is said, when and where, how he felt, and the names of any witnesses. He should also tell his teacher and school counselor and put that in writing as well. If the harassment continues, your teen can pursue legal remedies.

Situation:
You overhear your teen talking on the phone. She's asking the caller to please leave her alone. When you ask her about it later, you learn that she's been getting obscene phone calls.

Suggestions:
If she knows the identity of the caller, she should tell the person to stop. She should also tell the person how the calls make her feel. Ask

continued ➝

your teen to keep a detailed written account of the calls—when they are made, how often they are made, what is said, and how she feels. If she doesn't know the identity of the caller, report the problem to your telephone company or your local police. Ask them to help stop the offending calls. Meanwhile, tell your teen that she doesn't have to listen to the caller. She can just hang up.

GRAPHIC HARASSMENT

Sending certain types of pornographic material through the mail or over the Internet is illegal. Other sexually explicit materials—letters, photographs, magazines, videos, computer programs—may also constitute sexual harassment if they're repeatedly forced on people who don't want them.

Maybe someone keeps leaving obscene notes in your teen's locker. Maybe someone keeps showing your teen videos that include nudity and sexually explicit behavior, even though your teen has said he doesn't like them. Either could be a form of sexual harassment.

Tell your teen that whenever he is confronted with uninvited, unwanted, and unwelcome sexual material, he should make it clear that he finds it unacceptable. He might say something like, "Don't show me any more of those pictures. I don't want to see them. I think they're offensive." He can't expect the other people to read his mind; he needs to tell them clearly and directly what he thinks and how he feels. If the behavior continues, it constitutes harassment.

WHAT TO DO?

Situation:
You learn that your teen is upset because another student left pornographic pictures in her locker at school.

Suggestions:
Does she know who left the pictures? If so, she should tell the person to never do it again. She should explain that she finds such pictures offensive and it upsets her to see them. If the behavior continues, she should keep a detailed written account, save the pictures, then take them to the school counselor or principal, along with her written explanation. What if she doesn't know who left the pictures? She should take them straight to the counselor or principal.

continued →

> **Situation:**
> Someone is sending your teen pornographic pictures in emails.
>
> **Suggestions:**
> If this happens, your teen has several options. He can change his email address and only give it out to his closest friends. He can set up a filter on his email program that automatically sends email from the offender to a special folder, where it's easily deleted. He can contact your Internet Service Provider (ISP) and request that all emails from the offender be blocked. If the pictures keep arriving, have your teen save the emails, then contact your local police. In most cases, they will be able to locate the offender using information in the header of the email.

QUID PRO QUO HARASSMENT

Quid pro quo is a Latin phrase meaning "this for that." It's used to describe a deal in which both partners get something they want—as in "You scratch my back and I'll scratch yours."

Quid pro quo harassment occurs when someone suggests or demands sexual favors in return for something specific. A student who says "I won't tell anyone I saw you cheating on the test if you give me oral sex," or a teacher who says "I'll give you an A on your paper if you'll show me your breasts," is guilty of quid pro quo harassment.

Tell your teen that if something like this happens to her, she's not obliged to tell the abuser how she feels or warn him to stop. Quid pro quo harassment is illegal. She should inform you immediately, and you'll go together to the principal or the police.

ANTI-GAY HARASSMENT

Teens who are gay, lesbian, bisexual, or transgendered (GLBT)—or those who are assumed, accurately or not, to be GLBT—are often the brunt of jokes, teasing, name-calling, or outright physical assault. Gay bashing starts early, when kids use words and phrases like "fag," "dyke," "homo," "lezzie," "queer," and "that's so gay" without really grasping what they mean. As kids become teens, words can turn into threats, bullying, and violence.

Tell your teen that you expect him not to tell gay jokes. Explain that when he stays silent or laughs quietly when others tell them, he is giving indirect approval for these kinds of behaviors.

What if your teen tells you that people are teasing a friend of hers? Be clear about what you expect her to do. You might say, "When you hear someone teasing your friend for being a lesbian, I expect you to stick up for her."

What if your teen is afraid of being teased or labeled as a lesbian herself? You might say, "Behaving with integrity isn't easy, but it's worth it. Not only will you help your friend by sticking up for her, but you'll also feel good about yourself." Or "I understand how you feel. Sticking up for another person is always risky. But how will you feel if you stay silent? You're not the kind of person who stands by and lets other people be hurt. If you speak out, you may be teased or labeled, but you'll know you're doing the right thing."

JUST THE FACTS

■ In one study of students in public high schools, 97 percent reported regularly hearing anti-gay remarks from their peers.[7]

■ About two-thirds of gay students reported being physically or verbally harassed in school.[8]

■ Most young people who harass, bully, and assault GLBT people don't fit the stereotype of hate-filled extremists. They are average young people who often see nothing wrong with their behavior.[9]

What if you're the parent of a GLBT teen who experiences anti-gay harassment at school? We'll assume for the moment that you know about your teen's sexual orientation,* and that even if you don't approve, you love him and want him to be safe. Anti-gay harassment makes learning difficult for *all* students, not just those being harassed. And if your teen is being harassed, he's probably not the only one.

Under Title IX, the statute that bars sex discrimination in public schools receiving federal funds, anti-gay harassment that creates a sexually hostile school environment is illegal. Does that mean you should pursue legal remedies for your teen? Your decision will be based on many factors: what your teen wants, what you want for your family, how accepting the school is (or isn't) of GLBT students, and how accepting your community is, to name a few.

Some parents take legal action. Others talk to teachers and principals, explaining their concerns and asking them to be more aware and responsive. Some role-play possible strategies and responses with their teens. Others advise their teens to just walk away without reacting to the harassment, either verbally or physically.

Your teen will have to make his own choices about how to handle each incident. Meanwhile, you might find it helpful to connect with other parents of GLBT teens. Learn from each other what has and hasn't worked.

---

* See "Issue 3: Sexual Orientation" (pages 144–154).

Sexual Abuse and Sexual Assault

Sexual abuse is any form of sexual activity—including fondling, molestation, intercourse, and rape—committed on a child by a person responsible for the child's care, such as a parent, stepparent, day-care provider, or babysitter. Sexual assault is any form of sexual activity committed by someone other than a caregiver.

It's wrong to force *anyone* to engage in *any* form of sexual activity if the person is underage, doesn't understand what is happening, is under the influence of alcohol or drugs, or objects in any way. Make sure your teen understands that using physical, emotional, or psychological pressure to get someone to have sex is never acceptable. Neither are excuses like, "I was drunk," or "I was stoned, and I didn't know what I was doing," or "I thought he/she really wanted it." Emphasize that your teen is responsible for his or her own sexual behavior under *all* circumstances. Victims are the only exceptions to this rule.

INCEST

The family is supposed to be a safe place for children. Unfortunately, this is not the experience of teens who are subjected to sexual abuse by a family member.

If your teen tells you that a family member has been sexually inappropriate with him, listen carefully and take him seriously. Encourage him to talk freely. Reassure him that the abuse was not his fault, and that telling you was the right thing to do. Say that you will protect him, then follow through. Arrange for a medical examination. Report the abuse to your local Child Protection Agency.

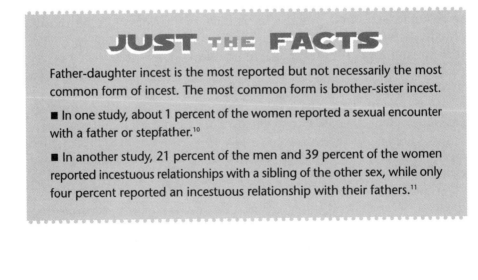

JUST THE FACTS

Father-daughter incest is the most reported but not necessarily the most common form of incest. The most common form is brother-sister incest.

■ In one study, about 1 percent of the women reported a sexual encounter with a father or stepfather.[10]

■ In another study, 21 percent of the men and 39 percent of the women reported incestuous relationships with a sibling of the other sex, while only four percent reported an incestuous relationship with their fathers.[11]

Some children and teens are afraid to tell anyone about the abuse. They're ashamed, confused, or terrified; some abusers threaten to hurt their victims even more or to harm other people they care about. Abuse victims may communicate in other ways—by trying to run away, attempting suicide, abusing alcohol and drugs, developing sleep problems, getting depressed, withdrawing from friends or family, becoming delinquent, or acting out.

If you learn or suspect that your teen has been abused, seek professional mental health assistance. Abuse can have serious long-term consequences. Children and teens need expert adult guidance to rebuild their self-esteem, cope with feelings of guilt and worthlessness, learn to protect themselves in the future, and overcome the trauma of being abused. The sooner help is made available, the sooner they can start to heal.

CRISIS HOTLINE

1-800-4-A-CHILD
(1-800-422-4453)

If you suspect child abuse or need help, call the Childhelp USA National Child Abuse Hotline. The hotline is staffed 24 hours a day, 7 days a week with professional crisis counselors. Anyone can call: abused children, troubled parents, individuals concerned that abuse is occurring, and others requesting child abuse information. For more information, visit the Web site at *www.childhelpusa.org*.

RAPE

The *first* thing a teen who has been raped needs is unconditional love. Any form of sexual abuse or assault can be a life-shattering event, and your teen needs your comfort and support above all else.

Some parents' initial response to a child's rape is shock, anger, and blame. "How could you have been so stupid?" "What were you thinking?" "Didn't I warn you?" Please keep those thoughts to yourself. Rape is devastating enough without parental judgment or disapproval. And the *last* thing a teen needs is to feel that she "deserved" to be raped, or that the rape was somehow her fault.

If your daughter is raped, take her to the nearest hospital emergency room immediately. You can call the police from there. Don't allow her to bathe, shower, change clothes, or even (if possible) urinate before going to the hospital. Any of these actions can destroy valuable physical evidence.

Tell your teen what will happen at the hospital. A doctor will examine her to check for injuries. A rape kit will be used to collect evidence, which may include clothing fibers, hairs, saliva, and semen. Photographs may be taken. A blood test and a cervical culture will check for pregnancy and STIs. You'll need to visit your teen's own doctor in a week or two to review the results of these tests and learn what, if anything, should be done next.

If your son is raped (yes, males can also be sexually assaulted), similar procedures will be followed.

JUST the FACTS

■ In one national study, about 9 percent of students in grades nine through twelve reported having been forced to have sexual intercourse. This included both male and female students, although it happened significantly more often to female students.[12]

■ Teens ages sixteen to nineteen are three and one-half times more likely than the general population to be victims of rape, attempted rape, or sexual assault.[13]

Many rape victims suffer from rape-related Post-Traumatic Stress Disorder (PTSD). Your teen will probably need counseling and emotional support after the rape. (You may need some, too.) There are organizations that provide specialized counseling. Many communities have rape crisis hotlines that will help you find resources close to you. Check the front of your local phone book under "Emergency Assistance" or "Community Service."

While you can't undo what happened to your teen, you can help with the healing process. Face this trauma together in a loving, supportive way.

CRISIS HOTLINE

1-800-656-HOPE
(1-800-656-4673)

The National Sexual Assault Hotline is operated by the Rape, Abuse & Incest National Network (RAINN), a nonprofit organization based in Washington, D.C. It offers free, confidential counseling and support 24 hours a day, 7 days a week. When a victim calls the

continued ➞

800-number, the call is immediately routed to the rape crisis center nearest the caller. RAINN has more than 1,000 crisis center affiliates across America. For more information, visit the Web site at *www.rainn.org.*

DATE RAPE

Date rape, also called acquaintance rape, is the most common form of rape today. Some people mistakenly believe that date rape isn't as serious as stranger rape, or even that it isn't "real" rape. But nobody asks or deserves to be raped. Nobody secretly wants to be raped. Rape is a felony crime, regardless of the offender's relationship to the victim. Date rape is every bit as devastating to the victim as stranger rape.

Talk with your teen about date rape and ways to protect herself. (Please note that, in spite of the pronouns used here, both girls and boys can be victimized.) Talk about how no means no.* Remind her that alcohol and drugs can impair her judgment, her communication skills, and her ability to determine whether a situation is safe or dangerous.**

Encourage her to be especially careful in group situations, where she might be pressured to do things she doesn't want to do. Tell her that if she ever feels threatened, she should state her position clearly (and loudly, if that's what it takes), then get away as soon as she can. Being embarrassed is better than being assaulted. If she's going to a party, she can make sure that friends she trusts will be there, too. They can agree to watch out for each other and keep each other safe.

Ask your teen if she knows about the so-called "date-rape" drugs. Rohypnol (also called Roofies, Rophies, and Lunch Money, to name just a few of its street names) and GHB (Grievous Bodily Harm, Liquid Ecstasy, Energy Drink, etc.) are colorless, odorless, and nearly tasteless. Either is easily added to a drink, where it's virtually undetectable. Either can cause dizziness, drowsiness, confusion, impaired judgment, and unconsciousness. Both are especially dangerous, and sometimes even fatal, when mixed with alcohol or drugs.

Date-rape drugs are impossible to detect but fairly easy to avoid. Tell your teen not to drink any beverages she doesn't open herself. To be on the safe side, she might even bring her own drinks to parties. Ask her not to exchange or share drinks, drink from a punch bowl, drink from a container that people are passing around, or leave her drink unattended for any amount of

---

* See also "No Means No" on pages 47–48.

** See also "Alcohol and Drugs" on pages 62–63.

time. If someone offers to buy her a drink at a party or club, she should watch it being made and carry it herself.

JUST THE FACTS

■ Seventy-seven percent of rapes are committed by people the victims know.[14]

■ One study found that 75 percent of the males and 50 percent of the females involved in college campus acquaintance rapes had been drinking.[15]

Abusive Relationships

As your teen begins to date, she may encounter a partner who misuses his position as an important person in her life. The partner may use his power over her to feel better about himself or manipulate her in order to get his way.

When your teen forms a relationship and starts seeing one person regularly, pay attention to how she behaves. Monitoring the way your teen and her partner make decisions can help you determine whether a problem exists.*

IS YOUR TEEN BEING ABUSED?

How can you tell if your teen's partner has crossed the line between being influential in your teen's life and being abusive? (Please note that, in spite of the pronouns used here, both girls and boys can be abused in either heterosexual or same-sex relationships.) Ask yourself these questions:**

- Is your teen frightened by her partner's temper?
- Is she afraid to disagree with her partner?
- Is she constantly apologizing for her partner's behavior?
- Does she have to justify everything she does to her partner?
- Does her partner try to control who she hangs out with?
- Does her partner put her down frequently yet tell her he loves her?
- Has she stopped seeing family or friends or stopped doing activities she used to enjoy just because her partner is jealous?
- Has she been forced into sexual activity she didn't want?
- Has her partner slapped or shoved her?
- Is she afraid to break up because her partner has threatened to hurt her or himself?

---

* See also "Dating" on pages 45–50.

** We are indebted to the New Jersey Department of Community Affairs, Office of Prevention of Violence Against Women, for some of the material in this and the following section.

If you answered yes to any of these questions, your teen may be on the receiving end of an abusive relationship. Don't let her delude herself that things will change, that her partner didn't really mean it, that he only acts this way because he loves her so much. Both your teen and her partner need help. If your teen is in this kind of relationship, she may have self-esteem issues that should be addressed professionally.

No matter what kind of pressure your teen feels, she can choose to end the relationship. This may be difficult, and she'll need your support and encouragement. If you're not sure what to do, consult her school's counseling department or a local crisis hotline. But do something. The situation is unlikely to get better, and it may get a lot worse.

IS YOUR TEEN ABUSIVE?

Do you think your teen may be abusing his partner? (Again, please note that, in spite of the pronouns used here, girls can be abusive to boys, boys can be abusive to boys, and girls can be abusive to girls.) Ask yourself these questions:

- Is he extremely jealous or possessive?
- Does he constantly check up on his partner?
- Does he continually accuse his partner of cheating on him, yet stay in the relationship?
- Has he ever hit, kicked, shoved, or thrown things at his partner?
- Does he constantly insult or criticize his partner?
- Does he become violent when he drinks or uses drugs?
- Has he ever threatened his partner or broken things in his partner's presence?
- Has he intimidated his partner so that she is afraid to say no to him?
- Has he threatened to hurt his partner?
- Has he threatened to hurt himself if his partner breaks up with him?

If you answered yes to even one of these questions, your teen's behavior is abusive. Once you recognize that a problem exists, get professional help for your teen. Talk with someone from your teen's school counseling department, consult your religious leader, or call a crisis hotline for information about local counseling options. But do something.

Don't try to justify your teen's behavior to yourself or to him. Don't make excuses for him, and don't let your teen blame his partner for what he's done. Make it clear that he's responsible for his own actions, and he needs help immediately. This is not a passing phase, and his abusive behavior won't just go away. Without intervention, it may escalate, and your teen could end up really hurting someone.

STALKING

What happens when affection turns into obsession? When a relationship ends, but one person won't let go? Your teen says her ex-boyfriend is following her, begging her to please get back together. The letters, the calls, and the emails won't stop. Recently they've become angry, harassing, even threatening. Yesterday, someone slashed her tires. Your teen is worried—and getting scared.

Stalking is illegal in all 50 states. If your daughter is being stalked, she may be able to get a restraining order against her former boyfriend. Depending on what has happened, she may be able to pursue other legal remedies.

Meanwhile, she should keep a detailed written account of all stalking-related incidents including phone calls, conversations, and threats. She should also keep anything that might be needed as evidence: answering machine or voicemail messages, letters, emails, photographs of property damage or other acts of vandalism. And she should tell as many people as she can about the problem—her friends, her teachers, her school counselors. They can help back up her story to the police.

Go with your teen to talk with a victim specialist, who can help you develop a safety plan. You'll find victim specialists at your local domestic violence or rape crisis program. Check the front of your local phone book under "Emergency Assistance" or "Community Service."

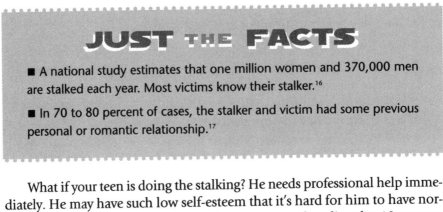

JUST THE FACTS

- A national study estimates that one million women and 370,000 men are stalked each year. Most victims know their stalker.[16]

- In 70 to 80 percent of cases, the stalker and victim had some previous personal or romantic relationship.[17]

What if your teen is doing the stalking? He needs professional help immediately. He may have such low self-esteem that it's hard for him to have normal, healthy relationships. He may have a personality disorder. No matter what the cause is, the stalking must stop.

Respect and Power

All the forms of sexual harassment and abuse described here are, in many ways, issues of respect—or the lack of respect. They all involve forcing one's will on another without regard for the other person's rights or feelings.

If your teen has experienced any form of harassment or abuse, try talking with her. Encourage her to share her feelings with you. It's common for abused people to blame themselves for the unwanted attention. They worry that they might have misinterpreted their abuser, or that they somehow deserved what happened to them. The abuser may have said things like, "The way you dress, you're asking for it," or "If you didn't want to have sex with me, you shouldn't have come here." Tell your teen that harassment and abuse are never the victim's fault.

Because sexual abuse is also about power, it can be difficult for your teen to confront her abuser. She may need your support to challenge the behavior of an authority figure. It's easy for teens to be intimidated by a person's position. Let your teen know that her body isn't community property, she has individual rights, and you'll be there for her and back her all the way.

It won't be easy for your teen to speak up, but doing so is her best defense. Sexual abusers not only lack respect for their victims. They also rely on their silence.

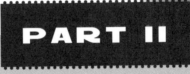

PART II

Issues to Know About and Talk About

FEMALE SEXUAL DEVELOPMENT

Wasn't it only yesterday that you held that little bundle of wonder in your arms? How could it possibly be that you're shopping for bras and talking about boys? When you were her age, the only "B" word you were thinking of was "bike" or "basketball." Isn't all this happening too soon?

Probably not. The average age of menarche, a woman's first menstrual cycle, has dropped to between twelve and thirteen.[1] While nobody is sure why this has happened, it's possible that improved health care, better nutrition, and advances in the control of infectious diseases all played a part. Your parents probably knew more about nutrition than their parents did, and when you became a parent, you had even better information. Whatever the reasons, children are physically maturing younger than they once did.

A Time of Change

Adolescence is all about change. Your daughter's body is slipping out of childhood and molding itself into a woman's. Sometimes the changes are slow; sometimes they are startling. When will these changes begin to take place? That's hard to answer, because everyone's body has its own built-in calendar.

Some of your daughter's friends may have been menstruating since the fourth or fifth grade; others may not begin until high school. Some girls her age have been wearing bras for months or years; others are still waiting for their breasts to develop. Reassure your daughter that her body is developing in a way that is natural and right for her.

If you haven't already talked with your daughter about the body changes of puberty, now would be a great time to start, especially if she's showing signs of entering puberty. You might want to say something like, "You're growing up, inside and out, and I'm proud of the way you're doing it." To a younger teen who hasn't yet shown the signs of puberty, you could say, "Soon your body will begin to change. It takes some time, but it's really exciting and

---

For practical reasons, we've divided female and male sexual development into separate chapters, but we suggest reading both, regardless of the sex of your teen. To be fully sexually informed, your teen will need to know about the sexual development of both males and females.

worth it." Then use the opportunity to talk in detail about the body changes she'll experience.

AVERAGE AGE AND AGE RANGE OF MAJOR PUBERTAL CHANGES IN NORTH AMERICAN GIRLS[2]		
	Average	**Range**
Breasts begin to bud	10	8–13
Height spurt begins	10	8–13
Pubic hair appears	10.5	8–14
Peak of strength spurt	11.6	9.5–14
Peak of height spurt	11.7	10–13.5
Menarche (first menstruation) occurs	12.8	10.5–15.5
Adult stature reached	13	10–16
Breast growth completed	14	10–16
Pubic hair growth completed	14.5	14–15

What you say and when you say it will depend on you and your teen. Talks about body changes can be separate from or combined with those about sexual expression. It's never too early to educate a child about her body parts. If you haven't mentioned terms like clitoris, ovaries, uterus, or hymen, you can start to use these words, always looking for real-life opportunities to begin conversations.

For example, when you see a pregnant woman, you might say, "Isn't it amazing that a woman's uterus can stretch enough to carry a baby?" Or "Did you know that a nonpregnant woman's uterus is about the size of your fist? Look at how big it can grow." Keep your information brief, and monitor your teen's reaction. Sexuality education is a lifelong process, not a one-time event, so you don't have to cover everything at once. If your teen seems interested and asks questions, continue. If she doesn't, drop the subject and bring it up again at another time.

You can use a noticeable change in a family member's or a friend's body to begin to describe breast development, the growth of pubic hair, and acne. Advertisements for soaps and deodorants also can be great jumping-off places for conversation. You might say, "Now that you're growing up, your body is changing and developing sweat glands, and you might want to try using a deodorant. We have some here already, or we can go shopping and try another brand if you want."

Your teen may want to know what causes all this change. Some of it is hereditary, but most of it is due to hormones.

Hormones: Nature's Chemical Messengers

Puberty, like many other biological processes, is supervised by hormones, the chemical substances that supervise many biological processes: growth, sexual development, blood pressure, metabolism. Like messengers, they travel from their headquarters via the blood to various parts of the body, carrying coded instructions for cells to react in certain ways.

When it's the right time for your daughter, her ovaries will begin to release female hormones called estrogen and progesterone into her bloodstream. These hormones will then travel to different parts of her body, bringing the message that it's time for her to start developing sexually.

One of the first signs that your daughter's sex hormones are on the loose is the budding of her breasts, followed by the appearance of hair under her arms and in her pubic area. At the same time, fat builds up under that hair on top of the pubic bone.

This raised area, with its upside-down triangle of pubic hair, is called the mons veneris, a Latin phrase meaning "mound of Venus" (Venus was the Roman goddess of love). That triangle makes the mons veneris stand out visually. Since a person's pubic hair is generally darker than the hair on her head, it seems to be nature's way of saying, "Here is an important place!" Perhaps that's why works of art, from prehistoric times to the present, have used a triangle to represent femininity.

The Perfect Body

Very few girls are happy with their bodies, and some go to extremes to bring themselves closer to the super-thin models and actresses they see. Teach your daughter about the dangers of extreme diets, and remind her that sexual attractiveness is as variable as the flavors of ice cream. For many people, sensitivity, kindness, and a willingness to share thoughts and feelings are more of a turn-on than having the "perfect" body. Sexiness comes more from what's on the inside than from what her body looks like on the outside.

If you feel that your daughter is too focused on her physical appearance, you might say, "It's great to work out, pay attention to what you eat, and keep your body looking good. But the right person will love you no matter what you look like." Or "How your body looks on the outside may be important to you. So take good care of your body, but don't overdo it. It's what's inside you that really counts."

The next time you're out in a crowd together, encourage your daughter to look around. Real women come in all shapes and sizes. There's no standard-issue female body, so it makes sense to help your daughter get comfortable with the one she has.

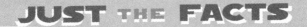

■ Eight million or more people in the United States have eating disorders. Seven million are women.[3]

■ Eating disorders usually start in adolescence, but they may begin as early as age ten or younger.[4]

The Breasts

Breasts begin to develop when fat cells migrate to their new home behind the nipples. Although it's more common for nipples to turn out, on some women one or both turn in. These are called inverted nipples, and they're a natural variation. If your daughter's nipples are inverted, assure her that she's fine. This doesn't mean that anything is wrong, or that she won't be able to nurse babies someday if she chooses.

During puberty, breasts become capable of feeding a baby. As a teen's breasts start to develop and swell, the area surrounding the nipple darkens. This area, called the areola, contains glands that can secrete a substance to help a nursing infant suck on a breast. When a woman nurses an infant, her nipples, which have lots of tiny holes in them, work something like a showerhead, letting the milk empty from her mammary glands.

Nipples are made of erectile tissue, which means they can get hard. This can be confusing and embarrassing for your teen. Explain that many things can cause nipples to get firm, and that sexual arousal is only one of them. Cold weather or the friction of an irritating fabric can do it, too. Assure her that it's perfectly normal and natural—every woman's body does it, and so do men's.

As your daughter's breasts continue to develop, she may find that one of them is growing faster than the other. Reassure her that the two sides of the human body are not perfectly symmetrical. For example, most people have one foot that's slightly larger than the other. Even if, right now, the difference between your teen's breasts seems conspicuous to her, it's probably so slight that other people won't notice it. Eventually, her breasts may even out.

Your daughter may have questions and concerns about the size of her breasts. Answer her questions honestly, and try to reassure her that her breasts are right for her.

WHAT TO SAY?

If your teen says . . .
"I can't go swimming. If I wear a bathing suit, everyone will see how lopsided I am."

You might say . . .
"Honey, trust me. No one will notice but you. Besides, it's normal. Human bodies aren't perfectly symmetrical."

If your teen says . . .
"I'm so flat-chested. Everyone has breasts but me."

You might say . . .
"Remember when you were little and you were upset because the tooth fairy had come to everyone's house but yours? Then your teeth started to fall out when they were good and ready. It's like that now. Your body is like nobody else's, and when it's good and ready, it will develop the right breasts for you."

If your teen says . . .
"I hate my breasts. Nobody else my age has them, and I'm sick of being teased."

You might say . . .
"It always hurts to be teased, but the other girls will develop breasts, too. You just started sooner."

If your teen says . . .
"I hate having a big chest. All the guys are always staring at me."

You might say . . .
"I understand how uncomfortable it can be to be stared at. If it really bothers you, let's come up with some things you might say to them." Then rehearse different responses she could give.

Teens don't always come right out and say what's bothering them. If you notice that your teen suddenly doesn't want to wear a bathing suit or always wears a sweater or an oversized jacket, you might want to check things out with her. You could say something like, "It seems to me that you're covering up your body a lot. Is everything okay?" Or "Are you okay with the changes going on with your body? Want to talk?" If you sense that something isn't right but she refuses to talk about it, you could say, "I know it's hard, but talking about what's bothering you, whatever it is, often helps. When you're ready, I'm here."

TOO BIG? TOO SMALL?

Breasts seem to come in two sizes: too big and too small. Few women seem to be satisfied with the size they actually have. Our culture has focused on breasts as sex symbols. Naturally, this makes women very conscious of the way their breasts measure up to some imagined ideal.

Women with smaller breasts may feel sexually inadequate. Your teen may have heard that small breasts are not as sexually sensitive, or she may be worried that she won't be able to breastfeed if and when she has children. Reassure her that neither sexual response nor the ability to nurse a baby are affected by breast size or shape. Size is simply a matter of how much fat is deposited behind the nipple.

If your daughter reads women's magazines, she'll probably see advertisements for devices, exercise systems, creams, and lotions that claim to increase the size of the breasts. Some devices and exercises can strengthen and develop the muscles that support the breasts, but they won't affect breast size. Creams and lotions may contain the hormone estrogen, but in such small amounts that their effect is insignificant. Tell your daughter that any and all of these products are a waste of her money.

The only proven way to increase breast size is breast augmentation surgery. Unfortunately, breast implants have become a hot trend among teens. What if your daughter announces that she wants implants? First, ask her why she wants them. Talk with her about body image, self-confidence, and self-esteem. Second, tell her that breast implants aren't a good idea when her body is still growing and changing. Even adult women can have complications from breast augmentation surgery, or problems later with the implants. Finally, you can tell your daughter that when she's an adult, she can make her own decision and have the surgery if she still wants to. By then, she might feel differently and be happy with her body the way it is.

JUST THE FACTS

In the year 2000, 212,500 women in America had breast augmentation surgery. Of these, 3,682 were teens age eighteen or under.[5]

Women with larger breasts may think they're "too fat," or they may feel that they're being stared at. If you sense that your daughter is uncomfortable with her breast size, you might say, "So many women waste time wishing they had larger or smaller breasts. Yours are right for you." Make sure that her bras fit correctly. A professional fitter at a major department store or lingerie store can help with this.

Regardless of her breast size, and despite what your daughter may have heard or seen in the movies, many women don't find that having their breasts touched is all that sexually exciting. That doesn't mean there's anything wrong with them, it just means that everyone's body responds differently to sexual stimuli. In some cultures, breasts aren't considered erotic at all—they're simply feeding stations for babies.

THE BREAST SELF-EXAM

Breast cancer is the most common form of cancer in women. Approximately one in eight women will develop this potentially fatal disease sometime in her life.[6] Men get breast cancer, too, but not as frequently as women. Because the risk of breast cancer rises with age, an adult woman is at greater risk than a teen, but teaching your teen how to examine her breasts now will get her into the habit.

There is no magic age when it's best to begin, but you can't start too early. Because children learn by the examples we set, any adult woman in your teen's life—mom, aunts, cousins, friends—should do routine breast self-exams. Make a pact to remind each other and your teen. Post the guidelines in a bathroom or on the refrigerator. Although some recent studies question the value of breast self-examination, it still seems to be the safest course.[7]

Suggest that your daughter get in the habit of examining her breasts once every month, at the same time in her menstrual cycle. Give her a copy of the guidelines on page 134. Explain that her menstrual cycle and hormones will change the sensitivity and configuration of her breasts, and that's why she should examine them at the same time each month. The best times to do a breast self-exam are right in the middle of her menstrual cycle or after she's finished menstruating. The only time that's not good is right before or early in her period, when hormones can make the breasts sensitive or cause them to become thicker.

When your daughter visits the gynecologist, the doctor will check her breasts for any changes. Some teens are embarrassed by the thought of a doctor examining their breasts. If your daughter is uncomfortable, reassure her that it's not a sexual touch. If she wants, she has the right to ask for a female nurse or assistant to be in the room with her during the examination, even if the doctor is a woman.

The Clitoris and the External Genitals

A woman's external genitals, the parts you can see, are called her vulva. The vulva is made up of the labia, the clitoris, and the vaginal and urinary openings.

Two sets of labia, or lips, protect the vaginal opening. The larger, outer lips—the labia majora—are composed of fatty tissue. As your daughter matures, they become covered with hair. The smaller, inner lips—the labia minora—are hairless and highly sexually sensitive in many women.

On top, just above the vaginal opening, the inner lips meet to form the clitoral hood. Under this fold of skin is the clitoris, a woman's most sensitive sexual organ. It has no other purpose than to provide sexual pleasure for a female. Unfortunately, in most sexual education courses, this organ is never even mentioned. In our opinion, saying nothing is a negative message. Not talking about the clitoris to your daughter or your son implies that women's sexual pleasure is not important.

How do you begin this discussion? You can start by adding the word clitoris to your vocabulary. When talking about sexual activity, many parents use the terms penis and vagina as though they were parallel organs. They're not. The clitoris, not the vagina, is the equivalent of the penis. Like the penis, it is an erectile organ that swells when aroused. If you have already used terms like penis and vagina while talking with your son or daughter, now say penis, vagina, and clitoris. The first time you do this, you may want to add, "The clitoris is that knob or button-like part just above the opening of the vagina. It's the place that's very sexually sensitive." Or you might say, "Women have something that's very much like a penis. It's called the clitoris, and it's located just before the opening to the vagina. It's very sexually sensitive and pleasing for a woman, just like a penis is for a man."

You might encourage your daughter to use a hand-held mirror to examine her external genitals. That's the best way to learn what the different parts look like on her own body.

Under the clitoral hood are glands that secrete a white substance called smegma, whose function isn't clearly understood. If allowed to build up, smegma can cause discomfort and even infection. Tell your daughter that when she's washing her vaginal area, she should clean gently and thoroughly around the clitoris and under the clitoral hood. She should use a mild, non-deodorant soap, since harsh or deodorant soaps can cause irritation.

The Hymen

Most females are born with a thin membrane called the hymen just inside the opening of the vagina. If it's still present, it usually tears the first time a female has sexual intercourse. That's what causes bleeding, if there is any.

In some ancient cultures, newlywed couples had to hang their sheets out after the wedding night for public inspection. Blood on the sheets was considered proof that the bride was a virgin before marriage. Some of these brides must have needed a trick or two, because not all women bleed the first time they have intercourse. The absence of the hymen doesn't mean a woman isn't a virgin. A woman can have a perforated or ruptured hymen for lots of reasons: a childhood accident, physical exertion, or even inserting a tampon, although using a tampon doesn't always tear the hymen.

Even if a woman's hymen is intact, she may not bleed noticeably when it's broken, although some women bleed a lot. It's another one of those things that differs from woman to woman.

A hymen is rarely a solid wall of membrane. It usually has one or more holes that allow menstrual fluids to flow out. So it's even possible, though unusual, to have intercourse without tearing it.

The idea of something inside them tearing and bleeding the first time they have intercourse makes many teens flinch. They expect it to hurt, but that doesn't necessarily happen. Tell your teen that if she's comfortable with her decision—if she's not worried about what her partner is going to think about her the next day, if she's not worried about getting pregnant or getting a sexually transmitted infection, if she's properly stimulated so that her vagina is well lubricated, if she's relaxed and feels safe with her partner, and if her partner is careful, thoughtful, and responsive to her needs—then her first (or any following) sexual intercourse doesn't have to hurt.

Your daughter and son will both need to know that when a man and a woman decide to engage in sexual intercourse, especially if it's the woman's first time, allowing the vagina to receive the penis slowly, with gentle pressure, is bound to be more pleasurable than just plowing on in.

The Vagina

The triangle of pubic hair frames the area of the vagina. Most people think of the vagina as a hole, tube, or tunnel. It isn't really any of those things. When it's at rest, the walls of the vagina touch each other, like the sides of a balloon when there's no air inside. But the vagina has an amazing ability to stretch to accommodate a tampon, a penis, or the passage of a baby.

The average vagina is three-and-a-half to five inches deep. Some young girls worry that their vagina will be too small for an erect penis, and some young men may worry that their penis, when erect, will be too large for the small opening they imagine the vagina to be. Let your teen know that a vagina is almost never too big or too small. It adjusts its size. When a woman is sexually excited, the back of her vagina spreads like a tent to make more room for a penis, in case intercourse does take place. If a man has an unusually long penis, some of it will just hang out.

You can tell your teen that vaginas are very smart. As soon as a woman becomes sexually aroused, her vagina starts to lubricate to prepare for the possibility of sexual intercourse. If a vagina receives a penis when it isn't lubricated, intercourse is uncomfortable or even painful. That's why making sure that a woman is sexually aroused is so important if sexual intercourse is to take place.

Advertisers try to persuade women, old and young, that they need to buy products that will make them "feel fresh." Unless a doctor tells her to, there's no reason for a teen or a woman to douche, or wash out the inside of her vagina. Douching needlessly can actually increase her chances of getting a vaginal infection. All she needs to do is wash her vulva daily with a mild soap.

The inside of the vagina keeps itself clean by secreting fluids, which change in consistency depending on where a woman is in her menstrual cycle. You may want to explain to your daughter that those fluids are what she finds on her underpants at the end of the day. It's nature's way of keeping the inside of her vagina clean and healthy.

Encourage your daughter to learn about her body, its fluids, and its changes so she'll know if something is ever wrong. For example, if vaginal discharge becomes thicker or changes in color, amount, or odor, it can signal an infection that may or may not have anything to do with sexual activity. Tell your daughter what you want her to do if she discovers a vaginal odor or change that doesn't go away in a day or so or after a shower or bath. Do you want her to tell you? Go to a doctor? Go to a clinic?

DOING THE KEGEL

In the 1940s, gynecologist Arnold Kegel discovered that women who had good muscle control over their pubococcygeus (PC) muscle were less likely to lose urine while coughing after childbirth, and that they experienced more intense orgasms. To strengthen the PC muscle, he developed an exercise now known as the Kegel.

Where is your PC muscle? The next time you urinate, start the flow and then stop it. If you're able to do that, you've found your PC muscle.

The Kegel exercise goes like this: Imagine that your bladder is full. Imagine that you've just sat down to void and the phone rings. Cut off your imaginary urine flow. Relax and imagine the flow continuing. Slowly, to the count of five, cut off the imaginary urine flow. Hold it, counting five. Slowly relax your PC muscle, counting five. Repeat this slow tensing, holding, and relaxing at least ten times, and do the whole set of ten exercises three times a day. Nobody but you will be able to tell when or whether you're doing it.

Tell your daughter about the Kegel exercise and how to do it. Explain that it may help prevent incontinence problems later in life, when and if she has children. If you want, you could mention that when she becomes sexually active, having a stronger PC muscle may make sexual intercourse even more enjoyable for her.

You might also tell your son that men with good PC-muscle control may last longer during intercourse. For a man to locate his PC muscle, he should see if he can move his erect penis up and down without touching it. (Teens sometimes call this doing chin-ups with their penis.) Once he's able to do this, he doesn't need an erection to exercise his PC muscle.

The Ovaries

Girls are born with two internal sex organs called ovaries. (Boys have testicles.) Both ovaries and testicles are gonads, or sex glands.

When your daughter was born, each of her ovaries already harbored 100,000 to 300,000 immature eggs, or ova. Although they are contained in tiny protective sacs, many of them died during her childhood. Maybe her brother or sister kicked her, or maybe she ran a high fever or fell off her bike. By the time a girl reaches puberty, each ovary has about 10,000–50,000 eggs left.

While only a small percentage of eggs survive, it's still a lot more than your daughter will ever need. The average woman matures only about 500 eggs in her lifetime, so nature has been more than generous.

When the sex hormones give the green light, an egg matures and bursts out of its sac. This process is called ovulation, from ovum, the Latin word for egg. The egg travels from the ovary to the uterus through a sort of long entrance hall called a fallopian tube. There is one tube for each ovary. Each is approximately four inches long. The inside is only about two human hairs wide.

Meanwhile, a woman's uterus has been busy preparing for the arrival of the egg. The uterus has an inner lining called the endometrium. Triggered by hormonal messages, the endometrium develops into a rich, spongy lining capable of supporting and nourishing a fertilized egg.

At this point, one of two things can happen. If sperm have been deposited in or near the vagina, they travel up the vagina into the uterus and then into the fallopian tubes, trying to fertilize the waiting egg. Although millions of sperm are present in the average man's semen, only one will have the honor of entering the egg cell. This process, called fertilization or conception, usually occurs in the first third of the fallopian tube. By the time the fertilized egg reaches the uterus, it has already started the early process of development.

If the egg is not fertilized, the thickened lining of the uterus, the endometrium, sloughs off and is discharged from the body. That discharge is part of menstruation.

Menstruation

Menstruation happens about 14 days after ovulation. As the endometrial lining breaks away from the uterus, some tiny capillaries open and bleed. Menstrual fluid is a combination of that blood—quite a small amount, actually—and the endometrial lining itself, which is a darker color.

Some teens worry because the flow at the beginning of their periods is brownish, but that's normal. A brown or blackish color usually indicates older blood. It means that the uterus started to bleed earlier, then stopped for some reason. As your daughter's period continues, she'll eventually flow red.

Some teens are concerned about the amount of blood they lose during their menstrual cycles. It may seem like a lot some days, but most women lose only two or three ounces of blood a month—about four to six tablespoons. A typical blood donor, by contrast, donates sixteen ounces of blood at a sitting.

Some teens aren't sure if they should use tampons. Your daughter may wonder if inserting a tampon means that she will no longer be a virgin. Explain that a virgin is someone who has never had sexual intercourse, and that inserting a tampon is not the same as having sex. It may tear the hymen, but that usually doesn't happen. And even if it does, your teen is still a virgin until she has had sexual intercourse.

Women should change their tampons frequently. A disease known as toxic shock syndrome (TSS) can be triggered by a tampon (or anything else) left in the vagina for too long. What's too long? Doctors differ, but it's generally believed that nothing—no tampon or contraceptive device—should be allowed to stay in the vagina for more than six to eight hours.

Teach your teen to wrap used tampons and sanitary napkins in toilet tissue, newspaper, or special bags made for that purpose and discard them in the trash. Flushing these products down toilets is bound to cause plumbing problems.

Although menstrual periods are sometimes called monthlies, and the menstrual cycle for many women is roughly a month, there's no exact length of time for the menstrual cycle. It's different for different women, and even for an individual woman at various times during her life. Any number of things can change the cycle, including stress, illness, intense exercise, or environmental factors. Even being around another woman who has a different menstrual cycle can cause your cycle to change, though nobody's quite sure why.

Some women experience premenstrual syndrome (PMS) a few days before they begin to menstruate. Common symptoms of PMS are bloating, tenderness of breasts, and irritability. Many treatments have been tried with varying degrees of success. Talk with your health care provider if you or your teen have been bothered by your teen's symptoms.

Although we know that ovulation usually occurs about fourteen days before menstruation, there's no sure way of calculating it in advance. It's unusual but entirely possible to ovulate during menstruation. Some young people think that they can't get pregnant if they have intercourse during a woman's period. Wrong! Unprotected sex always puts your teen at risk for pregnancy—and for sexually transmitted infections (STIs).

MENARCHE: A CAUSE FOR CELEBRATION

A girl's first period is often a very exciting time for her as well as for her parents. She's now a young woman. Some parents want to share this welcome news with their friends and relatives, but that might embarrass their daughter. If this is your impulse, check with your daughter first. Admit your own excitement: "I think it's wonderful. You're a woman now. It's the beginning of a new phase of your life." Then ask her how she feels. Would she object if you told other people? Be specific about which people, then respect her decision.

You may want to mark the advent of menarche with a special ceremony celebrating your daughter's transition into womanhood. You may want to take your daughter out to dinner at a special restaurant—one where parents don't usually bring their children. In some families, it's customary to give the newly menstruating girl a light tap on the face. The original reason might have been to scare away bad spirits or add color to a girl's cheeks. Whatever their origins, rituals help smooth the transition. It's nice to somehow communicate that coming into physical adulthood is special—worthy of note and celebration.

Some parents convey the message, by their tone and/or manner, that a menstruating woman should feel embarrassed or "unclean." For some girls, the only initiation they receive is a recitation of war stories: "You wouldn't believe the cramps I had when I was your age!" Calling menstruation "the curse" and "the plague" reinforce a negative expectation. Telling your daughter to hide her tampons or sanitary napkins where other family members won't see them can also send a negative message.

If your daughter is already menstruating, reflect for a moment on how you told her about menstruation. (Remember that sons need information about menstruation, too.) Did you explain what was going to happen, what it meant, and how she might feel? If you didn't, it's not too late. If you see an advertisement related to menstruation, use it as a teachable moment. You might say, "You know, we never talked about how you felt when you first got your period. What was it like for you?" You could also ask how she feels about it now. If your family never talked about this kind of thing when you were young, tell your teen that. Explain your discomfort, then say you'd like things to be different for her.

Some fathers greet this time in their daughters' lives as a signal to back away from physical displays of affection, perhaps out of fear that any touch will be misinterpreted as sexual. While any form of sexual contact between parent and child is always inappropriate, affectionate hugs, pats on the back, and kisses on the cheek are very much needed in all children's lives at every stage of their growth and development. Remember that the Child who lives inside your teen will always need a loving, protective, attentive father.*

MENSTRUAL CRAMPS

Your teen may experience cramps during menstruation. These cramps, called dysmenorrhea, come in two basic varieties.

Congestive dysmenorrhea, the most common type, is like traffic congestion. Instead of flowing smoothly, blood backs up in the uterus. It's quite

---

* See "The Miron Model" on pages 19–27.

common for women to have one or two days of heavier bleeding during a period. Sometimes, when the flow is heavy, blood accumulates in the uterus faster than it can exit. When blood pools, it can coagulate and form a clot. The uterus responds to those clots by contracting to push them out in the same way it would contract to expel a baby during labor. Those contractions are menstrual cramps. Because birth control pills often cause a lighter blood flow, which reduces the cramping, doctors sometimes prescribe them for severe cramping caused by congestive dysmenorrhea.

The other kind of dysmenorrhea occurs when the uterus pumps out too much of a particular kind of prostaglandin. Prostaglandins are chemicals that regulate the expansion and contraction of smooth muscles—the ones you can't control voluntarily, like your heart. Cramping caused by prostaglandins can be treated with antiprostaglandin medications, such as aspirin or ibuprofen. These products should only be taken with a physician's knowledge, never on an empty stomach, and only as needed. They can irritate the digestive tract and can even cause internal bleeding and other problems if not taken wisely.

There's no tried-and-true remedy for menstrual cramps. Exercise sometimes helps. A heating pad on the abdomen may help. If the flow is very heavy, ice on the abdomen may help. Suggest that your daughter experiment to find out what works for her. If these strategies don't work, ask her doctor for other suggestions.

MENSTRUAL MYTHS

Your daughter may hear one or more myths about menstruation. Examples:

- Don't wash your hair or get a permanent during your period.
- Don't bathe or swim during heavy flow days.
- Don't touch flowers—they'll wilt.
- Don't have sexual intercourse.
- Don't touch meat—it will spoil.
- Don't exercise.

Reassure her that these are nothing but myths. For most women, there's no medical reason to stop any kind of normal activity. A woman who's menstruating is basically no different from a woman who isn't.

The First Visit to the Gynecologist

Many health professionals recommend that young women start having regular gynecological checkups when they begin menstruating. Any woman who is thinking about becoming sexually active should certainly consult a gynecologist first to discuss birth control and ways to avoid STIs.

The idea of visiting a doctor who is going to look at and probe into her vagina may be distasteful and even frightening to your teen. With advance information and support from you, and with a sensitive and informed doctor, the exam shouldn't hurt or even cause her extreme embarrassment.

Explain to your daughter that the doctor will examine her both externally and internally. If she wants, she can ask to have a female nurse in the room during the exam. If your daughter's hymen is intact, the exam won't break it. Let the gynecologist know that this is your daughter's first exam. If your daughter feels frightened or awkward, tell her to say so. Most doctors will be sensitive to her needs and proceed with extra gentleness.

Some teens are afraid that they'll become sexually aroused when their genitals are manipulated, or that the doctor will be aroused by looking at them. Assure your daughter that there's nothing arousing about a gynecological exam—for the patient or for the doctor. Explain how important it is to see a gynecologist regularly. A doctor who knows her body well can help keep her healthy and assist her in making good sexual decisions—not just for now, but also for the future.

How to Do a Breast Self-Exam

1. Stand in front of a mirror with your hands at your sides. Look at your breasts and check for any irregularities, like dimples or swelling.

2. Raise your hands over your head and hold them there. Check to see if this causes any unusual or uneven changes in either breast.

3. Lie down flat on your bed. Put a pillow behind your right shoulder. Slide your right elbow up toward your head and put your right hand under your head. Put the four fingers of your left hand together and explore your right breast, firmly pressing and using a circular motion. After you've gone completely around the breast, spiral inward and circle the breast again until every part of the breast has been explored and you reach the nipple.

4. Move the pillow to behind your left shoulder. Examine your left breast using the four fingers on your right hand.

5. Sit up or stand up. Squeeze both nipples to see if any discharge occurs. If it does, or if you've felt any lumps, bumps, or thickening in either breast, see a doctor. Don't panic, though—lots of things can cause any of these symptoms, and they don't always indicate a cancerous or precancerous condition. Your doctor may order some simple tests that can help determine what's going on.

MALE SEXUAL DEVELOPMENT

Your son comes home, eats half the food in the refrigerator, then goes to his room and slams his door. You know something's bothering him, and after much coaxing, you learn that he's sick and tired of being so short. Even the girls in his class are taller than he is. And he's had it with his voice cracking every time he opens his mouth to say something. While a part of you might think this is all very sweet (your little boy is growing up!), it's obvious that your son is hurt and worried. What do you say?

Tell him that you understand how hard it must be. Remind him that girls generally start maturing a couple of years earlier than boys. Point out that most girls stop growing in their late teens, while boys often continue on into their early twenties. Say that everyone's body has its own internal clock, and some males mature earlier than others. Some of the kids in his class may be shaving by the time they start high school; others won't need to shave until much later. There's no way to slow puberty down or hurry it up. Eventually, physical maturity comes to everyone. Assure your son that when the time is right for his body, it will happen.

You might also want to remind him that his body is entering a phase of intense change, designed to transform him into a sexually mature male. Talk with him about these changes.

Active Hormones, Big Changes

Your son's puberty, the time in his life when he becomes able to reproduce, begins when his testicles begin to produce androgens, the male sex hormones. The principle one is called testosterone.

Hormones are chemical substances that supervise many biological processes: growth, sexual development, blood pressure, metabolism. Like messengers, they travel from their headquarters via the blood to various parts of the body, carrying coded instructions for cells to react in certain ways.

For practical reasons, we've divided female and male sexual development into separate chapters, but we suggest reading both, regardless of the sex of your teen. To be fully sexually informed, your teen will need to know about the sexual development of both males and females.

Among the first signs that your son's hormonal messengers have begun their job is the growth of his testicles. Each testicle is suspended by something called the spermatic cord. This cord allows the testicles to rise and fall, depending on things like temperature and sexual arousal. For many men, the left testicle ends up hanging lower than the right because of the somewhat longer left spermatic cord. Your teen might worry about this, so try to let him know before he starts developing sexually.

If you haven't yet talked with your son about the body changes accompanying puberty, you can use his growth spurt as an opportunity to start a discussion. When he starts to outgrow his shoes before they're even broken in, you might say something like, "Your testicles are going to look like an adult man's soon. As they grow, one might hang lower than the other." If he asks why, you might want to say, "It's nothing to worry about. It's just the way it is." Or "There's a cord that holds each testicle, and usually the one on the left is longer." Look for a teachable moment to talk with your daughter about testicles as well.

As your son's testicles continue to develop, hair grows on his scrotum (the pouch that contains his testicles), in the pubic area, and under his arms. For most boys of European descent, soft, downy hair, sometimes called peach fuzz, sprouts on their upper lip and lower face. The texture and amount of hair may differ according to a boy's racial heritage. Around the same time, his penis will begin to change in size and shape. Usually it gets longer first, then wider or thicker. Appearance of facial hair might be another opportunity to start a discussion about changes in his genitals.

Thanks to the traveling hormones, your son's larynx expands as well. The vocal cords and the larynx, which sit at the top of the trachea (the air passage from the back of the mouth to the lungs), make speech possible. As the larynx grows, it becomes visible as a bump in the throat, called the Adam's apple, and it alters the pitch of his voice, making it deeper. This often occurs slowly, which causes cracking, or sudden changes in pitch that embarrass many young men.

The Perfect Body

During puberty, your son will experience growth spurts that add inches to his height. It will probably take more time for his musculature to catch up. He may worry that he's too gangly and will never fill out. He may measure himself against some movie hero with rippling torso muscles and bulging biceps and begin working out with a vengeance.

While exercise is good for him, that doesn't mean he should spend endless hours at the gym trying to bulk up. Nor should he resort to steroids or other products that promise to transform him into a teenage Arnold Schwarzenegger. Most of these products don't deliver what they promise, and they can be hazardous to his health. Even over-the-counter supplements such as creatine and androstenedione ("andro"), while not steroids, may be unsafe.

JUST THE FACTS

■ Steroids are a special danger to adolescents. Even small doses can stop growth too soon. Adolescents may be at risk for becoming dependent on steroids. Adolescents who use steroids are also more likely to use other addictive drugs and alcohol.[1]

■ Some of the many possible side effects of steroid use include high blood pressure, heart disease, liver damage, cancers, blood clots, sleep problems, severe acne, baldness, reduced sperm count, impotence, aggressive behavior ("roid rage"), panic attacks, depression, and thoughts of suicide.[2]

AVERAGE AGE AND AGE RANGE OF MAJOR PUBERTAL CHANGES IN NORTH AMERICAN BOYS[3]

	Average	Range
Testes begin to enlarge	11.5	9.5–13.5
Pubic hair appears	12	10–15
Penis begins to enlarge	12	10.5–14.5
Height spurt begins	12.5	10.5–16
First ejaculation occurs	13	12–16
Peak of height spurt	14	12.5–15.5
Facial hair begins to grow	14	12.5–15.5
Voice begins to deepen	14	12.5–15.5
Penis growth completed	14.5	12.5–16
Peak of strength spurt	15.3	13–17
Adult stature reached	15.5	13.5–17.5
Pubic hair growth completed	15.5	14–17

What about eating disorders? Although this is more of a problem for girls, boys can also develop anorexia nervosa (starving themselves) or bulimia (bingeing and purging). Add these two disorders to the normal eating problems of teens—overeating, poor nutritional habits, and food fads—and it's evident that parents need to pay attention to how their sons are eating. Talk with your son about the importance of good nutrition and a balanced diet. If he's going to clean out the refrigerator three times a week, stock it with healthful foods.

Help your son understand that for actors whose careers depend on muscle definition, keeping their bodies in shape is a full-time job. They pay personal trainers and nutritionists handsomely to prepare them for their next superhero role. Explain that people are attracted to all different kinds of men, not just bodybuilders. Sexual attractiveness is as variable as the flavors of ice cream. For many people, sensitivity, kindness, and a willingness to share thoughts and feelings are more of a turn-on than muscles. Sexiness comes more from what's on the inside than from what his body looks like on the outside.

If you feel that your son is too focused on his physical appearance, you might say, "It's great to work out, pay attention to what you eat, and keep your body looking good. But the right person will love you no matter what you look like." Or "How your body looks on the outside may be important to you. So take good care of your body, but don't overdo it. It's what's inside you that really counts."

The next time you're out in a crowd together, encourage your son to look around. Real men come in all shapes and sizes. There's no standard-issue male body, so it makes sense to help your son get comfortable with the one he has.

The Perfect Penis

Few gardeners watch the growth of plants under their care with as much attention and anxiety as young men watch the development of their penis. If you ask their owners, almost every penis is too small. Real penises never seem to measure up to the perfect penis of a teen's imagination, which is fed by stories he's heard or images from X-rated movies and magazines.

While the size of flaccid (sexually unexcited) penises vary, most end up approximately the same size when erect. A penis that's small when soft tends to expand more than a larger one during erection.

JUST THE FACTS

■ A survey of 300 men done by Lifestyles Condom Co. in April 2001 found that the average length of the male sex organ when erect is 5.877 inches.[4]

■ Another condom company, Durex, surveyed 2,848 men and found that the average length of an erect penis is 6.4 inches.[5]

■ According to the results of an Internet survey, the majority of men have an erect size between 5.0 and 6.5 inches.[6]

If your son reads magazines aimed at men (which can include magazines on men's health and fitness), he'll probably see advertisements for certain products—herbal concoctions, pills, potions—that claim to enlarge the penis. These advertisements cater to the nearly universal male concern about size. Most of these products have no effect at all, and some can be dangerous.

Even if your son hasn't verbally expressed any concern, let him know that the perfect penis is just a male fantasy. You can't assume that silence means he isn't worried. You might initiate the conversation by saying something like, "Do the guys talk a lot about penis size?" Or "Are your friends making jokes about penis size? I hope you know that size doesn't really matter."

Your teen may have heard that you can tell the size of a man's penis by looking at the size of his feet, hands, or nose. There's no correlation between the size of the penis and any other part of the body.

Some teens have the idea that the bigger the penis a man has, the more satisfying a lover he will be. But sexual pleasure has more to do with the brain than the genitals. You might say something like, "You're going to hear all kinds of things about penis size and shape and pleasing a partner sexually. The truth is, pleasing a partner has little to do with your genitals. Good sex is about sharing and learning about each other."

The Real Penis

Like facial features or fingerprints, penises are unique to each individual, and they vary in appearance. Some are wider; some are longer; some have a larger tip, or glans. Some are circumcised, which means that the foreskin, a protective fold of skin covering the glans, has been removed.

Boys are often circumcised in infancy—sometimes for religious purposes, and sometimes because the parents believe it's more hygienic. If your son is not circumcised, he should pull his foreskin back gently and clean under it thoroughly when he showers. Beneath the foreskin are glands that emit a sticky substance called smegma, which may cause irritation or even disease if allowed to build up.

Some teens worry because their penis angles off to one side when erect. They're convinced they must have injured their penis somehow, perhaps by masturbating. It's a physiological fact that some erect penises tilt to the right or left, and this has no bearing whatsoever on health or sexual enjoyment. If your son is concerned about this, tell him that it's just the way his penis is, and it's right for him.

If he brings these concerns to you, great. That's a compliment on how comfortable he is talking with you about sexual issues. But many teens don't talk with their parents about what's bothering them, especially sexually. So it's up to you to initiate conversations with your son. Watch for teachable moments, like jokes on TV or in movies alluding to penis size or shape. Or you might start a conversation by saying, "Do guys still laugh and joke about penises getting broken or shaped funny because they've been masturbating too much? They did when I was growing up. I hope you know that some penises tilt to one side. There's nothing wrong with that. It's just the way it is."

Below the penis, in a sack called the scrotum, are a man's sex glands, or testicles. The testicles make the majority of the male sex hormones and also produce sperm cells.

Encourage your son to get to know what his penis, testicles, and scrotal sac feel like. Although it's not very common, cancer of the genitals does occur, and establishing good health habits early in life is important. Suggest that your son examine his genitals periodically for any unusual bumps, lumps, or growths that weren't there before. Tell him that the thickening he may feel at the top of each testicle is probably the epididymis, the storage tank for sperm, and it's perfectly normal.

The best time for a man to examine his testicles is after a hot bath or shower. The warm water relaxes the muscles and skin of the scrotum and allows the testicles to come down, or descend. Tell your son to gently roll each testicle between his fingers and his thumb until he's examined it thoroughly. All hard lumps and unusual developments he observes should be checked by a physician immediately.

Erection

Explaining the complex process of an erection—the swelling and enlargement of the penis—is an important part of any teen's sexuality education. An erection may be associated with a sexual response, but it may also happen for other reasons, especially in younger men. The rubbing of clothes, the body's natural sleep cycles, a fleeting thought—any and all can produce erections. They're a normal part of a healthy male's life, and they start while he's developing in his mother's uterus.

When an erection occurs unexpectedly, it can cause great embarrassment for a teen. Prepare your son for this and brainstorm ways to handle it. For example, if he can, he might go to the restroom until the erection subsides. Approaching this issue with a sense of humor may help, but teasing won't. If the Adolescent in you wants to play, this isn't the right time or the right topic.*

One popular slang word for an erect penis is "boner," even though there's no bone in the penis. When a male gets an erection, the arteries that bring blood into his penis open up, and the veins that carry the blood out close down, so blood can't leave the penis at the same rate that it's entering. It's like turning on the faucet of a bathtub and plugging the drain. The process is called vasocongestion.

The trapped blood collects in three holding chambers inside the penis. The two chambers on the top are called the corpora cavernosa. The one on

---

* See "The Miron Model" on pages 19–27.

the bottom, the corpus spongiosum, surrounds the urethra, which is the tube that carries either urine or semen, depending on the situation, from inside the body out through the penis. This may be economical, but it is potentially problematic, since urine is highly acidic and acids kill sperm.

Nature's solution to this problem is the Cowper's glands. During sexual arousal, these small glands, one on each side of the urethra, secrete an alkaline liquid known as pre-ejaculatory fluid. This neutralizes the acid in the urethra so most sperm can pass through unharmed. A male cannot feel the secretions of the Cowper's glands, and they may contain sperm. Explain this to your son and daughter so they both understand that withdrawal (pulling the penis out of the vagina before ejaculation) is not a safe method of birth control. Even if a male is able to withdraw from the vagina immediately before he ejaculates (and few young men can), the pre-ejaculatory fluid may be enough to get the female pregnant.

Semen

Sperm cells—the seeds that fertilize a woman's eggs at conception—are produced in a man's testicles, but they don't stay there long. The immature cells are sent to the epididymis, where they continue to develop and are stored. The epididymis, which is shaped like a Christmas stocking, sits on top of and wraps behind the testicle. Each testicle has its own epididymis.

When a man becomes sexually aroused, mature sperm cells leave the epididymis, travel through a long tube called the vas deferens and enter the urethra through the ejaculatory duct. At this point, sperm mix with fluids from the nearby prostate gland and seminal vesicles. This mixture of sperm and fluids make up semen.

The average ejaculation contains about a teaspoon of semen, but the amount will be different for different men—and also for the same man on different occasions, depending on his health, the amount of sexual stimulation, and the amount of time since he last ejaculated. Semen can also vary in consistency. When it first comes out of the penis, it's usually thick and sticky, but it liquefies within twenty minutes.

Some men have yellowish semen, some grayish, some almost white—it depends on the individual. If your son notices a change in the color of his semen along with symptoms like pain or burning when he urinates, he should be seen by a doctor. These may be signs of a urinary tract infection (which may have nothing to do with sexual activity), or they may be signs of a sexually transmitted infection.

Your son may wonder about prostate cancer. Maybe he's heard that a friend's father or grandfather has prostate cancer, or perhaps someone closer to home has recently been diagnosed. Like breast cancer in women, prostate cancer in men is a serious health concern. It's the second leading cause of cancer deaths in men.[7] Reassure your son that prostate cancer is not a young man's disease, is not related to sexual activity, and is not a sexually transmitted infection. Most men diagnosed with prostate cancer are over sixty. Between now and the time he reaches that age, there may be many medical advances for diagnosing, treating, and even preventing prostate cancer.

Ejaculation

Many males experience their first ejaculation during masturbation. They may have been masturbating for a while, and even experiencing orgasms, but without any emission of semen. And then suddenly, somewhere between the ages of eleven and fifteen, the fluids join the orgasm and they have an ejaculation.

During a sexual experience, sexual arousal and tension build. If stimulation continues, a male will experience an orgasm, which is a total body response. His muscles will contract, fingers curl, toes point, and a sudden release of sexual tension occurs. At the same time, a sexually mature man will usually expel semen.

While orgasm and ejaculation tend to occur simultaneously, they are two separate processes. One can occur without the other. In a sexually mature man, repeated acts of sexual activity that have included ejaculation may cause an orgasm without ejaculation, because he has temporarily used up his supply of semen. It's also possible, though rare, to experience ejaculation without orgasm (for example, in men with spinal cord injuries). If all this sounds complicated, that's because it is.

Before ejaculation occurs, the muscles at the bases of the bladder and the prostate close down to prevent urine from being expelled. Reassure your teen that he will not urinate during intercourse. The prostate, seminal vesicles, and part of the vas deferens contract, combining the fluids and the sperm to make semen, which is trapped in the urethral bulb. These contractions are experienced by a man as the point of no return.

The muscles that surround the urethral bulb and the base of the penis begin to contract rhythmically. These urethral bulb contractions propel the semen down through the urethra and out of the penis—ejaculation. This process repeats several times until all of the semen for this ejaculation has been expelled. Orgasm can continue beyond ejaculation if stimulation is maintained.

Preferably before he's old enough to ejaculate, talk with your son about ejaculation and semen, so he doesn't get worried or scared when it occurs. (Talk with your daughter, too.) Help your teen to have a positive attitude about normal body fluids. You might say, "Sometimes, after sexual stimulation, a fluid comes out of a man's penis. It's called semen." You can ease the discomfort and add a little humor by asking your teen to name the slang terms he's heard for semen. At some point, you'll want to explain that semen can carry sexually transmitted infections (STIs) from one partner to another.

Some teens think they're too young to get a girl pregnant if they've just started ejaculating, or if they haven't yet ejaculated. While it's true that adolescents' first ejaculations often contain no sperm cells, there's no guarantee of that. You might tell your teen, "Some kids think they can't get a girl pregnant because they've just started to ejaculate. That's not true." Or "I hope you know that if you can ejaculate, you can get a woman pregnant." If you want your son to remain abstinent (however you define abstinence), you might add, "That's one reason why I don't believe you should be having sexual intercourse." If responsible sexual behavior is your goal for your teen, you could say, "That's one reason why you should never have an act of unprotected sex—not until you're ready to take on the responsibilities of being a parent."

WET DREAMS

Some boys have their first ejaculation in the form of a nocturnal emission, or wet dream. Unless your son has already been told about the existence of semen, you can imagine his surprise when this gooey, sticky stuff starts shooting from his penis or he finds it on his pajamas in the morning. Should he tell anyone? What should he do with the wet pajamas or sheets? What's that unusual smell?

Explain that if he has a wet dream, there's nothing to be embarrassed about. It's just nature taking its course. It's not uncommon for males to have four to six erections during an eight-hour period of sleep. Because the penis extends from the body, it can be stimulated by unconscious movements during sleep—rubbing against the sheets, the bed, or pajamas. You might say, "Your body's telling you that you're starting to grow up. And I like the way you're doing it, inside and out."

You might tell your son that girls can also have sexual experiences during sleep. This doesn't seem to happen as frequently as wet dreams for boys, and there isn't any semen as evidence, but it does happen.

ISSUE 3

SEXUAL ORIENTATION

When parents imagine preparing their children for mature, responsible sexual relationships, most assume those relationships will be with partners of the other sex. That won't always be the case. Somewhere between two and twelve percent of all people are gay, lesbian, or bisexual.[1] Many experts believe that about ten percent of the U.S. population is primarily gay or lesbian.[2]

Maybe you know that your teen is gay. Maybe you think that he might be gay, or you wonder if he is. Even if you're 100 percent sure that he's not gay, he probably has important people in his life—friends, relatives, classmates, teammates, teachers, adult leaders—who are gay. Most families have at least one gay member in their extended family circle.[3]

The sexuality education of your teen should include conversations about sexual orientation. What you tell your teen will depend on your values and beliefs—like anything else you say about sexuality. The more positive, informative, and open you can be, the more your teen will learn from you. You might start by asking, "Do your friends ever talk about gays, lesbians, and bisexuals? What do they say?"

If you're a gay parent, you probably already talk with your teen about sexual orientation. Much of what we say in this chapter won't be news to you. We do assume that most of our readers will be heterosexual, if only because most of the population is heterosexual. But we hope you'll read this chapter anyway, because it may contain information that is helpful to you, too.

JUST THE FACTS

■ Researchers estimate that anywhere from six million to fourteen million children nationwide live with at least one gay parent.[4]

■ Children raised by gay or lesbian parents are no more likely to grow up gay or lesbian than other children.[5]

Defining Terms

Some people have romantic and sexual feelings primarily for people of the other sex. They are referred to as heterosexual, or straight.

Some people have romantic and sexual feelings primarily for people of their own sex. They are referred to as homosexual (both men and women), gay (usually men, sometimes both men and women), or lesbian (women only).

Some people are attracted to people of both sexes. They are referred to as bisexual, or bi.

Some people don't fit neatly into the first three categories. They may have characteristics, behaviors, and self-perceptions typical of, or more commonly associated with, persons of the other sex. They are broadly referred to as transgendered. These individuals may be transsexual—people who feel they were born into a body of the wrong physical sex and seek to do something about it, often by surgery or hormone therapies. Other terms used to describe transgendered people are bi-gendered, androgyne, drag queen, drag king, masculine woman, and feminine man. Transgendered people can be straight, gay, lesbian, or bisexual.

Some people are intersexed. They are born with physical characteristics that differ from what we expect males and females to have. In the past, intersexed people have been called hermaphrodites, but today that term is considered offensive and stigmatizing to many.

Some people aren't yet sure of their sexual orientation. They are referred to as questioning.

What about gender identity and gender roles? You may have heard those terms and wondered what they mean. Simply put, your gender identity is how you see yourself—as a man or a woman. Gender roles are the expectations our culture has of how men and women should look and behave, and the way we signal our maleness or femaleness to others. Gender identity is your subjective sense of being male or female. It's who you feel you are. Society can assign gender roles (what is masculine or feminine), but only individuals can determine their own gender identity.

JUST THE FACTS

■ According to the American Academy of Pediatrics, gender identity—the personal sense of one's integral maleness or femaleness—typically occurs by age three.[6]

■ Many gay men and lesbians report beginning to feel different from other children between the ages of six and twelve.[7]

Straight, gay, lesbian, bi, transgendered, intersexed, questioning . . . are you feeling at all confused? If so, imagine how an adolescent feels when most young people around her are starting to get interested in the other sex—and she's discovering her own attraction to people of the same sex. Meanwhile, she has already heard anti-gay slurs and homophobic remarks indicating that feelings like hers are different, unpopular, wrong, and even dangerous.*

To make things a little less confusing, we'll use GLBT (for Gay, Lesbian, Bisexual, Transgendered) to refer to people who aren't strictly heterosexual. Some people use LGBT, GLBTQ, and other combinations of letters, but GLBT appears to be the acronym most commonly found in the literature about sexual orientation, and it's the one used by many groups and organizations for gay teens and their families.

THE KINSEY SCALE

When trying to understand sexual orientation, many people find it helpful to think of heterosexuality, homosexuality, and bisexuality not as distinct categories, but as points on a continuum—a line with no clear divisions.

Alfred Kinsey, the renowned sexuality researcher, described sexual orientation using a scale from zero to six. On Kinsey's scale, a person at the zero end of the scale is exclusively heterosexual. All of his sexual thoughts, feelings, fantasies, and behaviors involve people of the other sex. A six is exclusively homosexual. A three is bisexual, with roughly equal heterosexual and homosexual thoughts, feelings, fantasies, and behaviors.

In his research, Kinsey found that zeroes and sixes are very rare. Most people are ones, twos, fours, or fives, meaning that they have at least some interest in the other sex *and* the same sex, whether or not they act on it.[8]

If your teen tells you that he has had sexual thoughts, dreams, or fantasies involving a person of the same sex, you might say, "Those kinds of thoughts, dreams, and fantasies are pretty common. A lot of people have them, including both straight people and gay people." Then you might explain the Kinsey scale to your teen.

Sexual Orientation—or Sexual Preference?

When talking with your teen about sexuality, which term should you use: sexual orientation or sexual preference? According to research, being gay, lesbian, bisexual, or transgendered is not a preference. Preference implies choice, and people don't choose to be GLBT. They can choose whether to act on their feelings, but they can't choose how they feel.

If people don't choose their sexual orientation, how does it happen? No one knows for sure, but most scientists today agree that sexual orientation

---

* See "Anti-Gay Harassment" on pages 108–109.

results from a complex interaction of environmental, cognitive, and biological factors. Recent evidence suggests that biology (including genetic or inborn hormonal factors) plays a major role.[9]

Sexual orientation doesn't equate to or predict sexual behavior. Many teens (and adults) may think of themselves as being homosexual or bisexual without ever having a same-sex relationship. Others may have same-sex experiences but identify as heterosexuals. Remember that adolescence is a time of seeking, exploration, and experimentation.

If your teen is GLBT, you can have the same general expectations for her sexual behavior as you would if she were straight. You can define your goals for her sexual behavior, then explain the model you want her to follow: abstinence, delayed sexual expression, or responsible sexual involvement.*

CAN PEOPLE CHANGE THEIR SEXUAL ORIENTATION?

You may have heard about something called "reparative therapy" or "transformational ministry."[10] Reparative therapy (also called conversion therapy) uses psychotherapy in an effort to eliminate homosexual desires. Transformational ministry uses religion. Both approaches assume that there is something wrong with homosexuality, and that it is a mental disorder that can and should be cured.

This view of homosexuality has been rejected by the American Academy of Pediatrics, the American Counseling Association, the American Psychiatric Association, the American Psychological Association, the National Association of School Psychologists, and the National Association of Social Workers. Together, these organizations represent more than 477,000 health and mental health professionals. Many believe that reparative therapy can seriously harm young people.

What about transformational ministry? Some congregations and conservative political organizations support the belief that "freedom from homosexuality" is possible through faith and repentance. This view is not shared by all people of faith. Many deeply religious people and many congregations and denominations are supportive and accepting of GLBT people and their right to be protected from discrimination and harm.

If your teen is concerned, confused, or uncertain about her sexual orientation, counseling may help her sort out her feelings. Check out the counselor's views ahead of time. In its policy statement on homosexuality and adolescence, the American Academy of Pediatrics notes that "therapy directed specifically at changing sexual orientation is contraindicated, since it can provoke guilt and anxiety while having little or no potential for achieving change in orientation."[11] If you believe that your teen would benefit from talking with a religious leader, find out first where that leader stands on the issues.

---

* See "Step 5: Choose Your Model and Customize It" (pages 60–75).

What If Your Teen Is Questioning?

You're talking with your teen about sexual orientation when she mentions that she sometimes wonders about herself. Don't jump to conclusions—either way. You could say, "A big part of being your age is discovering your sexual orientation. It's not unusual to be confused. You'll figure it out with time. If talking helps, I'm here."

If you already leave sexual information (books, pamphlets, videos, etc.) out in the open for your teen to find, you might also make information available about sexual orientation. This lets your teen know that she doesn't have to sneak around or feel ashamed if she wants to know more. It also gives you some control over the sources she turns to for information.

If your teen says, "I think I'm gay," find out what she knows about homosexuality and why she thinks as she does. In our practice, we've seen young men who think they're gay because they're not athletic, they love ballet, or they cry easily. Some young women have questioned their sexual orientation because they hate wearing dresses or makeup, or they're more interested in football than cooking. We've also seen teens who think they're gay because they've engaged in some sexual experimentation with a friend of the same sex, or because they're attracted to a new student teacher who is the same sex they are.

Some of these teens were gay; others were not. Masculinity and femininity have little to do with sexual orientation. Also, sexual orientation is not determined by isolated sexual acts, but by consistent patterns of sexual behavior.

What If Your Teen Is Gay?

"Mom, Dad, I have something to tell you. I'm gay."

Most parents aren't prepared to hear those words—even parents who consider themselves to be open, informed, and accepting. Your first thought might be, "Oh, no!" or "How could he do this to me?" or "How will I handle this?" or "What did I do to deserve this?" or "What did I do wrong?" Or maybe, "I've lost my child forever."

Try to keep those thoughts to yourself. Your teen has just taken a big risk by coming out to you—by identifying himself as gay. This signals his confidence and trust in you. He probably knows that many gay teens are rejected by their parents. He hears anti-gay language every day at school. He may be aware that many gay teens experience harassment, threats, and violence, and some eventually decide that life isn't worth living.

JUST THE FACTS

- Each year, an estimated 125,000 homeless teenagers identify themselves as gay or lesbian. Half of them (almost 63,000) say they were thrown out of their homes by their parents because of their sexual orientation.[13]

- The typical high-school student hears anti-gay slurs 25.5 times a day.[14]

- Gay adolescents are more than two times as likely to attempt suicide as their heterosexual peers.[15]

What should you say? That depends on you. First, try to understand that you haven't lost your child. You've lost your image and dreams of your child. He's the same person he was five minutes ago, before he came out. He hasn't changed. You may see him very differently now, but that's because you know something about him that you didn't know before.

Then look inside your heart. Speak from the best in you to the best in him. Maybe all you can say at the moment is something like this: "Thank you for being honest with me. I know it must have been hard for you. Right now, I'm not sure what to say. I need some time to think. Meanwhile, I want you to know that I love you."

WHAT NEXT?

Families vary as much in their acceptance of homosexuality as they do in their feelings about sex before marriage. Much of how you react to your teen's coming out will depend on your own values and beliefs. But there are some things we hope you'll consider, no matter what.

Continue showing your teen love and support. He's still your child. Never forget that. Some of the problems parents (and people in general) have with GLBT teens start when they focus on the "sexual" part of "homosexual" (or "bisexual") as the main issue. Stop for a moment and think of your own romantic relationship. It's not just about sex. Neither are romantic relationships among gay men, lesbian women, or bisexuals.

Some heterosexual parents have a very hard time accepting that their child is GLBT. If you're one of them, try to figure out why you feel that way. Some reasons are selfish in nature: "Now there's no one to carry on the family name," or "What will I tell the neighbors?" or "I'll never have grandchildren," or "This isn't the lifestyle I want for my child." These thoughts don't come from your Adult.* Other reactions are based on concern and do come from your Adult: "I don't want my teen to have a hard life," or "I worry about HIV/AIDS," or "Will he ever be happy?" or "I'm afraid that he'll be teased, harassed, or a victim of hate crimes."

While there is no way to address all of these issues here, we can offer some suggestions. First, try not to put your concerns, whatever they may be, on your teen's shoulders. Instead, be available. Ask him how he's feeling. Ask how you can help. The truth is, this is not your issue. It's your teen's issue. Have faith in his ability to create a happy, fulfilling life for himself.

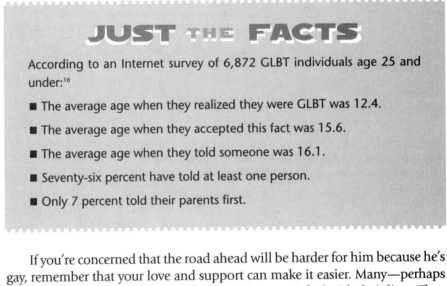

JUST THE FACTS

According to an Internet survey of 6,872 GLBT individuals age 25 and under:[16]

- The average age when they realized they were GLBT was 12.4.

- The average age when they accepted this fact was 15.6.

- The average age when they told someone was 16.1.

- Seventy-six percent have told at least one person.

- Only 7 percent told their parents first.

If you're concerned that the road ahead will be harder for him because he's gay, remember that your love and support can make it easier. Many—perhaps most—gay, lesbian, and bisexual individuals are satisfied with their lives. They may struggle to come to terms with their sexual orientation, and they often experience discrimination. But the road ahead might not be as hard for your child as you think. Many GLBT people find strong, supportive communities and form tightly knit circles of friends—"families of choice." Often, these circles of friends expand to include straight friends and family members. Many parents become even closer to their children than they were before.

We've talked with parents who felt they'd failed or done something wrong because their teen is GLBT. What's important is not what you did or didn't do, which had little or no influence on your teen's sexual orientation anyway. What's important is what you do from now on. Can you accept your teen? Support your teen? Communicate the message that his sexual orientation is normal and natural? Be part of his life, even though it may not be the

---

* See "The Miron Model" on pages 19–27.

life you once imagined for him? Set aside any prejudices and misconceptions? Advocate for him? Going forward, that's what matters most.

Some parents are concerned about the legal implications of being GLBT. While there is nothing illegal about being gay, certain sexual behaviors that many GLBT (and heterosexual) people engage in are technically illegal in many states. These laws are enforced very rarely these days—but when they are, enforcement is often selectively used against homosexuals. You might want to learn the laws in your state that pertain to sexual behavior. Meanwhile, know that most GLBT individuals live their lives without ever having problems with the police or the legal system.

Because being gay, lesbian, bisexual, or transgendered is seldom talked about in positive terms, and because there are relatively few positive role models and social supports, many young GLBT teens struggle with their sexual feelings in isolation. Talking with your teen and keeping the lines of communication open can help prevent this.

How will your teen adjust to the realization that he's gay? That varies tremendously from teen to teen. Some embrace their sexual orientation, making the adjustment quickly and contentedly. Others try to hide from it by aggressively pursuing activities they associate with heterosexuality. Boys may go out for sports; girls may act more "feminine" or become shy and withdrawn. Both may try heterosexual dating. Some lesbian teens may become pregnant; some gay male teens may try to get a girl pregnant. Still others escape into alcohol and drugs. And some get so depressed that they become suicidal.*

Your support, understanding, and acceptance can make a big difference in how successfully your teen adjusts—to being himself.

Try This

Fold a piece of paper in half. On the top of one side, write "Female." On the top of the other side, write "Male." Now write every term you've ever heard used to describe male and female homosexuals. All levels of language are acceptable here. Afterward, look at what you've written. What kinds of words do you see? Are any of them positive?

BE INFORMED

We've all been conditioned to view homosexuality in negative terms. We know the stereotypes: that gay men are limp-wristed and effeminate; that

---

* See "Depression" on pages 57–59 for warning signs and crisis hotlines.

lesbians wear flannel, have short hair, drive trucks, and hate men. We've heard the myths: that all gay men are HIV-positive and most are child molesters; that gays try to influence (or "recruit") young people; that being GLBT automatically means you'll have problems and be unhappy.

GLBT teens learn those negative words before they discover their own sexual orientation. That's one of many reasons why some GLBT teens have difficulty forming a positive self-image.

Being a minority is always challenging. Being GLBT in a heterosexual world can be especially difficult. When African American, Latino, Asian, Jewish, or Islamic children experience prejudice, they can go home to their families and find comfort, familiarity, and support. Their family members are usually of the same minority. But GLBT teens often don't have that solace. They are usually born into families where the parents are heterosexual, as are most (if not all) other family members. By coming out, they risk losing their families' affection. Some are rejected by their friends. Suddenly, they're isolated and alone.

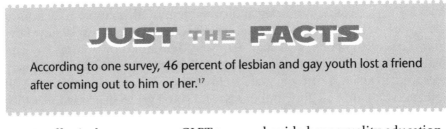

JUST THE FACTS

According to one survey, 46 percent of lesbian and gay youth lost a friend after coming out to him or her.[17]

To effectively parent your GLBT teen and guide her sexuality education, you'll need to set aside the stereotypes, ignore the myths, and get answers to the many questions you may have about homosexuality. Keep an open mind. Be curious. Learn as much as you can. Read books and magazines. Contact national organizations and request information. Go online.*

GET CONNECTED

When your GLBT teen comes out to you, it's possible that *you'll* feel isolated and alone. Who can you talk to? Who can you trust? You worry what other people might think and say—maybe even your own partner. You fear that the news will upset your parents—your teen's grandparents.

Sometimes our fears are worse than reality. Many parents of GLBT teens don't tell other family members for years. When they finally do, they often hear, "What took you so long to tell us? We've known about it for ages."

One of the best things you can do for yourself—and your teen—is to talk with other parents of GLBT teens. They've been where you are now. You're not alone.

---

* See "Resources" (pages 228–238) for many excellent sources of information.

Do's and Don'ts for Families and Friends

Do listen to what your loved one's life is like, and what kind of experiences he or she has had in the world.	**Don't** blame your own feelings on your loved one.
Do take the time to seek information about the lives of GLBT people from parents of GLBT people, friends of your loved one, literature, and, most of all, directly from your loved one.	**Don't** rush the process of trying to understand your loved one's sexuality or gender identity.
Do get professional help for anyone in the family, including yourself, who becomes severely depressed over your loved one's sexuality or gender identity.	**Don't** assume that your loved one should see a professional counselor.
Do accept that you are responsible for your negative reactions.	**Don't** criticize your loved one for being different.
Do help your child (or loved one) set individual goals, even though these may differ drastically from your own.	**Don't** expect your child (or loved one) to make up for your own failures in life.
Do try to develop trust and openness by allowing your loved one to choose his or her own lifestyle.	**Don't** try to force your loved one to conform to your ideas of proper sexual behavior.
Do be proud of your loved one's capacity for having loving relationships.	**Don't** blame yourself because your loved one is gay, lesbian, bisexual or transgendered.
Do look for the injured feelings underneath the anger and respond to them.	**Don't** demand that your child (or loved one) live up to what your idea of what a man or woman should be.
Do defend him or her against discrimination.	**Don't** discriminate against your loved one.
Do respect your loved one's right to find out how to choose the right person to love and how to make relationships last.	**Don't** try to break up loving relationships.
Do say, "I love you."	**Don't** insist that your morality is the only right one.

ONE PLACE TO TURN

PFLAG (Parents, Families and Friends of Lesbians and Gays) is a national nonprofit organization with over 200,000 members and supporters and nearly 500 affiliates in the United States. Their mission is to promote the health and well-being of GLBT persons, their families, friends through support, education, and advocacy. It provides opportunities for dialogue about sexual orientation and gender identity, and acts to create a society that is healthy and respectful of human diversity. Call, write, or go online to learn more, read or request some of PFLAG's many publications, and find a chapter near you.

PFLAG
1726 M Street NW, Suite 400
Washington, DC 20036
(202) 467-8180
www.pflag.org

SEXUAL EXPRESSION

Sexual expression is a natural part of growing up, an essential part of normal human development. Whether you want your teen to be abstinent until marriage (however you define abstinence), to delay sexual expression until some later landmark, or to participate responsibly in some forms of sexual expression,* he needs a well-balanced grounding in all types of sexual information.

Talking about the dangers of sexual behavior without discussing its pleasures is like describing the high fat and caloric content of chocolate without explaining how good it tastes. If you prepare your teen by sharing your values and by giving him solid information on various sexual behaviors, he can make positive, healthy choices for himself when he begins to be sexually active.

Remember that in communication, it's not only what you say, but how you say it.** Always try to be aware of who's doing the talking—your Child, your Adolescent, or your Adult.***

What Is Sex?

You've talked with your teen about why you feel she should wait to have sex until she's married, in a committed relationship, or at least older (much older). Or you've talked with her about what you believe responsible sexual involvement means. You've listened as she shared her thoughts and feelings, and you know that she wants to save sex for the right person at the right time. While you and she may not be in complete agreement about who that person will be and when that time will happen, you're reasonably confident that you understand each other.

Right?

Not exactly, because what sex means to you and what it means to your teen may be very different.

---

* See "What Do You Want Your Teen to Do—or Not Do?" on pages 66–69.

** See "Building Communication Skills" on pages 80–86.

*** See "The Miron Model" on pages 19–27.

When most parents talk with young people about sex, they're thinking about penis-and-vagina sexual intercourse, not oral sex, anal sex, mutual masturbation, or same-sex activity. Similarly, most of the research on adolescent sexuality (what little research there is) focuses on intercourse, not other forms of sexual expression.

The federal government has been reluctant to sponsor research into the full range of sexual behaviors among adolescents. Any research on teen sexuality not directly linked to teen pregnancy sparks conflict. Questions about behaviors "beyond" intercourse are considered taboo. There's the widespread belief that asking teens about sex somehow encourages them to be sexually active. Also, the research that is done almost always assumes that teens are heterosexual, effectively ignoring the sexual activities of gay, lesbian, bisexual, or transgendered (GLBT) teens. So while there's a lot of anecdotal evidence about what teens are and aren't doing sexually, there's not much hard data available.

But there is some. According to a 1994 survey, more than half of teenagers remain virgins until they are at least seventeen.[1] In a more recent (1996) study of urban high school students in grades nine through twelve, 47 percent reported being virgins.[2] Those numbers are meaningful only if we know how teens define words like "virgin" and "abstinence."

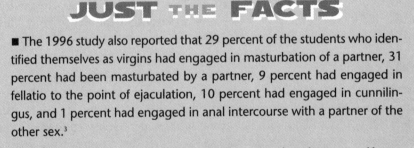

JUST THE FACTS

■ The 1996 study also reported that 29 percent of the students who identified themselves as virgins had engaged in masturbation of a partner, 31 percent had been masturbated by a partner, 9 percent had engaged in fellatio to the point of ejaculation, 10 percent had engaged in cunnilingus, and 1 percent had engaged in anal intercourse with a partner of the other sex.[3]

■ In a 1994–1995 survey of college freshmen and sophomores, 61 percent considered mutual masturbation to be abstinent behavior, 37 percent described oral sex as abstinence, and 24 percent thought the same about anal intercourse.[4]

■ In a fall 1999 survey of fifteen- to nineteen-year-olds conducted by *seventeen* magazine, 49 percent of teens considered oral sex to be "not as big a deal as sexual intercourse," and 40 percent said it did not count as sex.[5]

■ In a summer 2000 Internet survey conducted by *Twist* magazine, 18 percent of thirteen- to nineteen-year-old girls said that oral sex was something you did with your boyfriend before you are ready to have sex.[6]

Many teens who consider themselves virgins are, in fact, sexually experienced. So what, exactly, do being a virgin and having sex mean? Before you discuss these issues with your teen, you'll need to resolve these questions in your own mind.

From your perspective, is kissing having sex? Does it matter what kind of kissing it is? Are people having sex when they fondle breasts? When they stimulate the other person's genitals with their hands? With their mouths? What about anal sex? Are people having sex if a partner doesn't ejaculate or reach orgasm? If the partners reach orgasm but one person's genitals never actually touch the other person's genitals, as in rubbing bodies together or masturbating in the presence of a partner, is that sex? Do your answers change when they're applied to males instead of females? Once you've answered these difficult questions for yourself, approach your teen and explore some of the same ideas together.

Try This

Ask your teen to "just suppose" that her best friend, a virgin, recently confided that she kissed someone—really kissed someone. Does your teen feel that the friend and her partner had sex? Does she think that her friend is still a virgin?

Continue asking "just suppose" questions about sexual activities. Encourage your teen to add questions of her own. For each activity, ask:

1. Did your friend have sex?

2. Is your friend still a virgin?

Just suppose your friend told you that . . .

- her partner fondled her breasts through her clothes
- her partner felt her breasts under her clothes
- she touched and played with her partner's genitals
- she masturbated her partner to orgasm with her hand
- she touched her partner's genitals with her mouth, but there was no orgasm
- she used her mouth to stimulate her partner's genitals to orgasm
- her partner's hand masturbated her to orgasm
- her partner's mouth touched her genitals, but there was no orgasm

continued ⟶

- her partner's mouth stimulated her genitals to orgasm
- she had anal intercourse that didn't lead to orgasm
- she had anal intercourse that led to orgasm

Why separate sexual behaviors that lead to orgasm from those that don't? Because many teens believe that the latter "don't count" as having sex.

Once you've explored these issues with your teen, ask her to "just suppose" that her best friend is a boy. Then rephrase the questions and ask them again. (Example: "Just suppose your friend told you that he fondled his partner's breasts through her clothes. Did your friend have sex? Is he still a virgin?")

Ask your teen to give reasons for her answers. When you disagree, don't let your Child or Adolescent say, "That's wrong!" or "I can't believe you feel that way!" or "How could you say that?" Instead, have your Adult respond with questions like, "Why do you think that?" "Do your friends see it that way, too?" "I don't understand the distinction you're making. Could you tell me more?"

Tell your teen exactly what you think having sex and being a virgin mean. Be straightforward and nonjudgmental. Tell her why you think and feel as you do. You might say, "I don't agree with you about that," and then explain why.

Masturbation

Masturbation can be a normal, healthy way for teens (and adults) to express their sexuality, learn about their own sexual responses, and release sexual tension. Although there is no medical or psychological reason to refrain from masturbation, some people's religious, moral, or personal values prohibit or discourage it.

Share your values on this topic with your teen. If you believe that masturbation is wrong, you might say, "You're going to hear that it's okay to masturbate, but I don't think it is because . . . ." If you believe that masturbation is acceptable, say so explicitly, since it's often the topic of teasing and jokes.

Masturbation is very difficult for many people to talk about. This may have something to do with the myths and misinformation that have circulated for a long time. Many people once believed (and some still believe) that masturbation led to hairy palms, warts, blindness, stunted growth, stunted genitals, insanity, and other grisly consequences. Many religions had (and some still have) prohibitions against masturbation. In the late 1800s and early 1900s, some medical professionals taught that masturbation caused many ills.

Because of the hush-hush atmosphere surrounding masturbation, young people often get the impression that they're the only ones who enjoy this secret pleasure. They may be worried, embarrassed, and reluctant to bring up the topic. That's why it's your job to initiate the discussion. If you have difficulty talking about masturbation, join the club. Masturbation seems to be the most difficult sex-related topic to talk about, even among married couples.

Try This

Here's a way to ease some of your discomfort around the topic of masturbation. Pick a time when nobody else is around your house, then stand or sit in front of a mirror. Now whisper the word *masturbation* ten times. Are you still breathing? Say "masturbation" ten times in your regular speaking voice. You haven't fainted yet? Shout MASTURBATION ten times. See? You didn't die of embarrassment after all.

Now choose someone with whom you can repeat this exercise. It can be a partner, parent, or best friend. Explain the exercise, do it together, and follow up with a conversation about why the topic of masturbation makes you so uneasy.

Try to figure out where your discomfort is coming from. Is it your Child? Your Adolescent? Perhaps your Adult needs to have an internal dialogue with those parts of you and help them get a bit more comfortable.

If you wait for the media to provide you with a teachable moment—a TV program, movie, or advertisement about or alluding to masturbation—you'll wait for a very long time. Rape, sexual infidelity, child sexual abuse, sexually transmitted infections (STIs), and violence (both sexual and not) are all portrayed in prime-time TV programs and movies, but masturbation is seldom mentioned. (Exceptions: the *Seinfeld* "Master of My Domain" episode and the *American Pie* movies.) Chances are, you're going to have to start the conversation yourself.

While we don't recommend that you grill your teen about his masturbatory activities, you could ask something like, "Do the kids in your class make jokes about masturbation?" Then ask, "Why do you think they do?"

You may want to point out that jokes are one way to deal with things that people aren't comfortable talking about. Now that you've opened the door, you have the opportunity to share your values and listen to your teen's.

Try This

Here's an exercise you can do with your teen (and other members of the family, if you wish). Write down all the words and phrases for masturbation you can think of. Tell your teen that any kind of language is acceptable here. You'll probably get some laughs out of this, but you may also get good insights. If your teen is anything like the teens we work with, you'll end up with a long list of words that are male-oriented, regardless of your teen's sex.

Explore what messages the words and phrases convey. You might point out that women also masturbate, even though there aren't as many female-oriented words for it. Why the lack of language? Is it because women don't talk about masturbation as often as men do? Maybe. Why don't women talk about it? Ask your teen's opinion.

This exercise can also be a chance to look at the double standard that still exists when it comes to sexual expression: Sexual activity is okay for men, but not for women. You might discuss whether this is biologically determined (because of the sudden high levels of testosterone in adolescence) or socially determined (we expect men to be more sexual). You might ask your teen if he agrees with the double standard and why. Expect some interesting conversations.

Preparing your daughter for her period offers a great opportunity to talk with her about masturbation. While explaining menstruation, you might say, "The hormones that cause all this also create sexual feelings. Everyone has them, and they're natural." If you think that masturbation is sinful or wrong, you could add, "It's okay to have sexual feelings, but it's not okay to touch your clitoris or vagina when you do." Or "Sexual feelings will come and go. I believe that you shouldn't masturbate to relieve them." If you think that masturbation is okay, you might say, "Stimulating your clitoris and vulva will feel good and relieve sexual tension."

For your son, buying yet another new pair of jeans to fit his growing body could be an opportunity to start a conversation on masturbation, as could finding sheets or pajamas that are semen-stained from either nocturnal emissions or masturbation. You might say, "The same hormones that are causing your body to grow are also going to cause sexual feelings." If you think that masturbation is okay, you could add, "As your body grows and experiences sexual feelings, masturbation is a safe way to explore your body and learn about what's sexually pleasing to you." If he looks uncomfortable or seems embarrassed, you could say, "There's nothing to be embarrassed or ashamed about. Ejaculating is just a natural thing your body does, like breathing." You might also want to tell him what you want him to do with his pajamas or sheets.

If masturbation is not consistent with your beliefs, then the stained sheets or pajamas are still a good opportunity to present your position. You might start by saying, "Wet dreams are inevitable and nothing to worry about. It's just nature's way of exercising your body and getting it ready for when you're older. However, if ejaculation was brought on by masturbation, I have a problem with that." Then explain why.

JUST THE FACTS

■ More men than women talk about masturbation. Men report masturbating three times more frequently than women during early adolescence and young adulthood.[7]

■ Researchers have found no links between adolescent masturbation and early sexual activity (for example, frequency of intercourse, number of different partners, or age at which one has first intercourse) or sexual adjustment during young adulthood.[8]

DEBUNKING MASTURBATION MYTHS

Myths about masturbation still abound, and your teen has probably heard at least some of them. They might not be as lurid as the ones your great-grandparents heard, but they can be just as worrisome to a teen. Reassure your teen that all the myths she heard are simply that—myths.

Some myths begin in childhood. It's not uncommon for parents, frustrated by a child's persistence in rubbing her genitals inappropriately, to say something like, "Stop playing with yourself!" Your teen's "self" is a lot more than her genitals. If you're not happy with messages you gave your child in the past, now is a good time to correct any misinformation.

Where to start? You might use various springboards to begin a discussion about things that happened when she was little. Perhaps you're reminiscing about when she began playing soccer or doing gymnastics. From there, you can branch off into explaining that you were frustrated by her masturbating and you didn't know how to deal with it. You might say, "You know, we've both grown up a lot. I remember that I told you [whatever you said about masturbation at the time]. You know that's not true, don't you?" Then turn the conversation toward what you think is and isn't okay now.

Let your teen know that other people can't tell just by looking at her whether she has masturbated. It won't cause dark circles under her eyes from fatigue. If anything, it may help her to relax. It won't cause acne or loss of concentration. It won't affect her studies or her athletic or school performance.

Some teens worry that masturbation will change the size or shape of their penis, clitoris, or other body part. It won't. Some boys fear that if they masturbate too much, they'll use up all their semen. But once a boy's body starts producing semen, it will continue to do so throughout his life, and he can't possibly use it all up. He might, however, experience an orgasm without ejaculation. If a male ejaculates frequently within a relatively short period of time, he can temporarily diminish his semen supply. Tell your teen that if this happens, his body will soon create more semen.

Teens sometimes worry that if they spend too much time (whatever that means) masturbating, they won't be able to enjoy sex with a partner. Wrong again. Masturbation is not a substitute for sexual activity with a partner. It's just a different way of experiencing sexual pleasure. In fact, studies have shown that women who are able to masturbate to orgasm are much more likely to be orgasmic in a relationship.[9] When a woman knows from self-stimulation and experimentation what an orgasm feels like, it's easier for her to experience one with a partner.

For both sexes, masturbation can build sexual self-awareness and self-confidence. As long as masturbation isn't isolating your teen or taking her away from appropriate friends and tasks, she's fine. Some teens don't masturbate at all, and that's okay, too. It's a personal thing.

A few cautions are useful, however. Teens should know:

- to keep their hands clean
- to be careful not to introduce feces into the vaginal or urethral areas
- not to use sharp objects; anything that comes in contact with the genitals should be clean and smooth
- to use a water-based lubricant (if they like the feel of a lubricant) and avoid oil- or petroleum-based products such as hand lotion, baby oil, and petroleum jelly

The spread of STIs has given rise to another myth: that masturbation actually causes them. If your teen wonders out loud about this, don't laugh. Simply say, "A sexually transmitted infection is given by one person to another during sexual activity. You can't give yourself a sexually transmitted infection if you don't already have one."

MUTUAL MASTURBATION

Some couples engage in mutual masturbation, which means that they masturbate each other or themselves in each other's presence. This can be an expression of deep intimacy and an enjoyable way to release sexual tension.

If you believe that masturbation is okay if done in private—to oneself, by oneself—but that mutual masturbation is not okay for your teen, make a clear distinction between the two. For example, you might say, "I think it's okay for you to masturbate, but I don't think a partner should touch or see your genitals until [you're married, older, in a committed relationship, finished with high school, on your own financially, or whatever]."

In deciding whether mutual masturbation is an acceptable sexual behavior for your teen, remember that there's good and bad in almost everything. On the positive side, mutual masturbation reduces sexual tension with no risk of pregnancy or STIs as long as no body fluids are exchanged. It may also be a safe way for your teen to learn about sexual responses. On the negative side, it may be against your moral or religious beliefs, it may carry the risk of one partner not respecting the limits that both partners have previously agreed to, and it may lead to riskier behaviors, such as unprotected sexual intercourse.

You might want to share this list of positives and negatives with your teen. You could even ask if he has something to add to the list.

Outercourse

Outercourse is any sexual behavior that does not include oral, anal, or vaginal penetration or contact with semen, vaginal fluids, or blood. It includes things like hugging, caressing, sharing sexual fantasies, and massage—all lower-risk ways of finding sexual pleasure that stop short of actual intercourse or the sharing of body fluids. Slow dancing, rubbing bodies together, masturbation, mutual masturbation, and using sex toys* can also be considered forms of outercourse because no body fluids are exchanged.

Why talk with your teen about outercourse? Because it's one way to explain that a lot of sexually satisfying behaviors don't include sexual intercourse or the exchange of body fluids. If you want your teen to delay sexual intercourse, it might help to offer positive alternatives.

Television and movies can provide teachable moments. You can wait until you see some form of outercourse (you probably won't have to wait long) and say, "That's one type of outercourse." If your teen asks, "What's outercourse?" you might say, "It's any form of sexual expression that doesn't include intercourse or the exchange of body fluids." Then go on to discuss your views on outercourse and ask about his.

---

* See "Sex Toys" on pages 216–217.

You can also begin a conversation with a question like, "Have you ever heard the word outercourse?" If he hasn't, explain what it means. You and your teen can also make a list (spoken or written) of all the behaviors that would fall under that heading. Then present your values on each behavior and listen to his.

When discussing outercourse, mutual masturbation, or any shared sexual behavior, you'll also want to talk with your teen about respecting a partner's comfort level and boundaries. Teach him that no means no* and stop means stop—no matter how sexually aroused either partner might be.

Teachable moments about respecting boundaries occur frequently in families. For example, you might observe your teen teasing a younger sibling who says, "Stop!" or "Cut it out!" That's an opportunity to remind your teen to be respectful—of his siblings and everyone else.

Oral Sex

Whether you like it or not, whether you are comfortable with it or not, it's important to talk with your teen about oral sex.

The technical names for oral sex are fellatio (oral stimulation of the male genitals) and cunnilingus (oral stimulation of the clitoris and vulva). When both are done at the same time, it's referred to in slang terms as sixty-nine (69), because that number looks a bit like two people engaging in oral sex with each other.

You may be thinking, "That's all very interesting, but *my* teen would *never* have oral sex!" Maybe you're right—and maybe you're wrong.

The *Washington Post, New York Times, USA Today,* and *Talk* magazine, among others, have reported that increasing numbers of adolescents are engaging in oral sex as early as middle school. According to twelve- to sixteen-year-olds interviewed for *Talk,* seventh grade is the starting point for oral sex. By tenth grade, they say, more than half of their classmates are involved.[10]

These reports are anecdotal—they're not scientific. For reasons given earlier, there's been very little research into adolescent sexual behavior that's not directly related to teen pregnancy. We can't be sure if oral sex is really more common today among adolescents than it used to be, or if teens are simply talking about it more. Either way, this topic should be part of your teen's sexuality education. Most sex education courses don't cover it, so it's up to you to tell your teen about the possible consequences of oral sex.

While many parents consider oral sex an extremely intimate activity, teens often don't. According to one sexuality educator at a Baltimore school, some middle-school girls see it as a "bargain."[11] They stay virgins, they don't

---

* See also "No Means No" on pages 47–48.

get pregnant, and they think they can't get STIs. In fact, many STIs can be transmitted by either fellatio or cunnilingus, including human papillomavirus (HPV), herpes, hepatitis B, syphilis, gonorrhea, chlamydia, chancroid, and even (though rarely) the human immunodeficiency virus (HIV, the cause of AIDS).[12]

Unlike sexual intercourse, which teens frequently describe as something boys do to girls, fellatio is something girls can do to boys and remain in control. But is it really control, or is it exploitation? What if girls are performing oral sex on boys because they're being pressured, coerced, or forced, because they're afraid they won't be popular if they don't do it, or because they think they have to do it in order for boys to like them? Girls seem less likely to allow boys to perform oral sex on them. This may be due to how girls feel about their bodies. Many girls and women have a less than positive view of their genitals.

Tell your teen that vaginal secretions and semen can pass STIs. To avoid this, partners should use a latex condom over the penis during fellatio, or a latex film like a dental dam over the vulva during cunnilingus. If a dental dam is not available but a male condom is, they can unroll the condom, cut it lengthwise, and place it over the vulva. If a female condom is available, they can cut it along the seam and place it over the vulva.

Some experts believe that plastic food wrap can also be used to cover the penis or vulva during oral sex. There is some controversy over whether microwaveable plastic wrap should be used—do the tiny holes that let out the steam also let in STIs?—but warnings against microwaveable wrap are often dismissed as rumors. Plastic bags, "baggies," and trash bags should not be used, since they are weaker than plastic wrap.[13]

Fellatio and cunnilingus are technically illegal in many states, even if both people are consenting adults. These laws are rarely enforced, however, especially if the behavior does not occur in a public place.

You can explain to your teen that the decision to engage in oral sex is a personal matter and depends on individual values. Encourage her to not let herself be pressured into doing something she's not comfortable with. Give your views on oral sex and ask about hers.

If you believe that oral sex is an acceptable alternative to intercourse, you might say, "Oral sex is a form of sexual expression that can provide pleasure for both partners. You can't get pregnant, but you can get a sexually transmitted infection, so always protect yourself and your partner by using a latex condom or dental dam." Some parents think that oral sex is okay, but not for teens. If you share this view, you might say, "I think that oral sex is something very special and should be saved for [whatever you think is the right time or situation]."

Some parents are concerned that one sexual behavior will lead to another. If this worries you, you might say, "Oral sex when you're married is fine. When you're not, it could easily lead to other behaviors that aren't okay. I think it's better to be safe than sorry." If you believe that oral sex is not acceptable under any circumstances, you might say, "I think that oral sex is not okay for you or anyone." If you have moral or religious concerns about oral sex, explain them.

If you know or suspect that your teen's friends are beginning to engage in oral sex and you don't agree with this behavior, you might say, "Lots of your friends might be doing lots of things I don't agree with. I hope you're going to be true to what you believe is right." Adding "I believe in you" might help, too. Remember that the Child inside your teen still seeks your approval. In any dialogue with your teen, communicate what you think is or isn't okay and why.

Your teen may wonder about the "right" way to give oral sex. If she asks, you might say, "There isn't any formula for giving (or receiving) oral sex, but you don't want your teeth to come in contact with your partner's genitals. That can hurt. Everyone is different sexually, so it's a good idea to talk with your partner about what he or she finds pleasurable."

Your teen may have questions about the taste, consistency, or smell of semen or vaginal secretions. You might say, "It's a matter of personal likes and dislikes. Many people find the sight, smell, and taste of their partner's genitals highly erotic. Others don't. What's right for you may be different from what's right for someone else."

Teens often wonder about what to do with the ejaculate or semen. If your teen asks, you could say, "If you ever decide to have oral sex, use a condom and you won't have to worry about that. People who are monogamous and have been tested for sexually transmitted infections can either spit it out or swallow it, or they can pull away before their partner ejaculates." You may want to emphasize again that semen and vaginal fluids can transmit STIs, adding, "Unless your partner has been tested and hasn't had an act of unprotected sex since that test, you can't know for sure if he has a sexually transmitted infection. That's why you should always use a latex condom."

Anal Sex

People have varying feelings and beliefs about anal sex. Whatever values you hold, it's important to share them with your teen, along with the information she needs to keep herself healthy.

Teens need to know that anal sex poses health risks, both from STIs and from infections caused by transferring bacteria to the vaginal or urethral areas. Anal sex is illegal in many states, although the laws are rarely enforced.

Explain to your teen that because the anal area doesn't lubricate, the inner lining of the rectum is more likely to tear, making a person more vulnerable to an STI if her partner carries one. If your teen chooses to engage in anal sex, she should use lots of water-based lubricant on a latex condom. Anything that enters the anus should be introduced slowly and gently, allowing the anal sphincter to relax, or damage may be done to the anal area.

Caution your teen to never let anything that has come in contact with the anus or rectal area touch the vagina or the clitoris. The bacteria that live in the anal area are hostile to the vaginal and urethral areas and can cause infections. Whatever has come in contact with the anal area must be washed well with soap and water before ever being introduced into the vaginal area. It's okay to go from the vaginal area to the anal region, but not to do the reverse.

Sexual Intercourse

A general definition of sexual intercourse is "putting the penis inside another person's body." If the penis goes into the vagina, it's vaginal intercourse. If it goes into the mouth, it's oral intercourse. If it goes into the anus, it's anal intercourse.

Sexual intercourse is not exclusively heterosexual, although that's how many people define it. Some people who are GLBT prefer the term sexual activity over sexual intercourse, or they use other terms that avoid the assumption of heterosexuality.

By this point, we hope you're feeling more comfortable with the language that describes the mechanics of sexual intercourse. You can probably say words like erection, clitoris, penis, and vagina to your teen without getting tongue-tied. If you can't, you might return to the "Try This" activity on page 160. Instead of saying masturbation, substitute the word(s) you're having trouble with.

Once you've discussed your values about sexual intercourse with your teen, explaining the facts is relatively easy. You can say things like, "When a woman becomes sexually aroused, her vagina lubricates. If they decide to have intercourse, it feels good for both her and her partner." Similarly, you can say, "When a man becomes sexually aroused, his penis becomes hard, or erect." Or "When both the woman and man are ready, the vagina can receive the penis, which can feel really good for both partners." Remind your teen to always protect himself and his partner from STIs and pregnancy.*

Teens often worry about the "first time," and your teen may have lots of questions. Be as open and honest with your answers as you can.**

---

* See "Issue 5: Safer Sex" (pages 170–205).

** See "Issue 6: Sexual Pleasure" (pages 206–217) for more detailed answers to questions your teen may have about arousal, foreplay, and orgasm.

WHAT TO SAY?

If your teen asks . . .
"Will it hurt [me/my partner]?"

You might say . . .
"The human body is made for sexual intercourse. If it weren't, nobody would be here. So you can relax. If your mind is okay with what your body is doing, you'll be fine."

You might add . . .
"If you and your partner are comfortable with your decision and you're protecting yourselves from pregnancy and sexually transmitted infections, you can relax and enjoy this special act. If you're not emotionally ready, or you're worrying about any of the consequences, you may be tense. Putting anything—a tampon, a finger, a penis—in a vagina that's tense could hurt."

If your teen asks . . .
"How do I know if I'm ready?"

You might say . . .
"There's a whole list of things you can check for. Make sure you're not trying to prove your love for your partner, get attention, patch up a relationship that's falling apart, prove that you're mature, be like your friends, or rebel. Ask yourself how you'll feel the next day."

You might add . . .
"Be sure you're not just responding to pressure. If your partner is ready but you're not sure, wait. Take time to talk with your partner about what having sexual intercourse means to both of you. Talk about sexually transmitted infections and birth control. For intercourse to be a good experience, you both must be ready. You're going to remember your first time for the rest of your life."

If your teen asks . . .
"How can I make sure my partner has an orgasm?"

You might say . . .
"You can't. Each person is responsible for his own sexual response. But you can talk with your partner and find out what he likes and how he likes it. That will increase the chances that you both experience orgasm."

continued ➔

> **If your teen asks . . .**
> "What if my [vagina/penis] is too small?"
>
> **You might say . . .**
> "Sex isn't only about vaginas and penises. Those parts of the body are almost always the right size. Your mind is your most important sex organ. If you're both ready emotionally, you'll provide pleasure for yourself and your partner."
>
> If your teen doesn't ask any questions about the first time, you can. You might ask something like, "How do you want to feel after you've had sexual intercourse for the first time?"

Look for opportunities to talk about the joy of sex in a long-term committed relationship—perhaps seeing an older couple holding hands. Help your teen understand that shared sex in a monogamous relationship doesn't have to become boring. We human beings can be creative with our sexuality. Experimenting with a partner can be fun.

You might explain that during sex play or intercourse, either partner can be on top, or the couple may have intercourse nestled together like spoons. Sexual expression can happen in a bed, on the sofa, or anywhere in the house. People can be incredibly inventive about finding new positions, new forms of expression, and new ways of providing mutual pleasure with the same partner—for a lifetime.

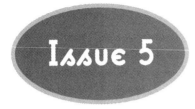

SAFER SEX

For many of us, life seemed easier when our children were young. True, we had to worry about our little ones running headlong into the street or eating their toys, but it beat worrying about pregnancy and sexually transmitted infections (STIs). Trying to keep your children safe while they develop sexually isn't easy, but someone has to do it, and that someone is you.

JUST THE FACTS

Only 11 percent of teens get most of their information about STIs from parents and other family members.[1]

Giving your teen sound, factual information is one of the most important ways to ensure her safety.* You won't be present when most dangers present themselves. Your teen must learn to anticipate the consequences of her actions, and know exactly what those consequences might be—for the short term and the long term. That's not an easy task at any age. In the world of sexuality, the lack of knowledge can be life-changing and even deadly.

JUST THE FACTS

■ Every year, three million teens—about one in four sexually active teens—acquire an STI.[2]

■ In a single act of unprotected sex with an infected partner, a teenage girl has a 1 percent risk of acquiring HIV, a 30 percent risk of getting genital herpes, and a 50 percent chance of contracting gonorrhea.[3]

---

* This chapter includes information you may want to share with your teen. See "Resources" (pages 228–238) for many excellent sources of additional information.

- In some studies, up to 15 percent of sexually active teenage girls have been found to be infected with human papillomavirus (HPV). Many are infected with a strain linked to cervical cancer.[4]

- A sexually active teenage girl who does not use contraceptives has a 90 percent chance of becoming pregnant within one year.[5]

- In a study of 650 girls age fourteen to nineteen who attended clinics in a large city, 40 percent were found to have an STI at the first visit.[6]

Why "Safer" Sex?

Totally safe sex is an unattainable ideal, like noncaloric chocolate. No sexual activity with a partner is entirely risk-free. That's why we use the phrase "safer sex" instead of "safe sex."

Safer sex is sexual activity that involves simple, practical precautions. It presents almost no risk of acquiring or transmitting infections or getting injured.

Many parents fear that talking with their teens about safer sex sends the message that being sexually active is okay, even when that's not what they mean. Study after study confirms that giving teens this information doesn't encourage them to start having sexual intercourse, increase the frequency of intercourse, or increase their number of sexual partners.[7] A lack of information may prevent them from making positive, healthy decisions about sexual expression.

JUST THE FACTS

According to a national survey, teens want to know more about STIs, how they are spread, and how people are tested for them. They want to know more about the various kinds of contraception and where to get contraception. They also want to know more about how to bring up STIs and birth control with a boyfriend or girlfriend.[8]

You might start by saying something like, "You know that I feel very strongly that you should wait [until you're married, or much older, or whatever you believe] to have sexual intercourse or engage in other sexual behaviors, like oral sex. But it's important for you to learn about safer sex practices now, so you're ready when you do become sexually active. That's why we need to talk about the risks of sexual activity, and how you can protect your-self and your partner."

Give your teen a copy of "What's Your Risk?" on page 201. This simple questionnaire lets your teen know immediately if he may be at risk of acquiring an STI. Because honesty often depends on confidentiality, don't insist that he share his finished questionnaire with you. Do encourage him to come to you if he has any questions or concerns.

Sexually Transmitted Infections

Sexually transmitted infections (STIs) are spread by sexual contact through semen and vaginal secretions. Blood and breast milk can also transmit the organisms that can cause infections. So can contact with an open sore. STIs can be passed from a mother to her baby before, during, or immediately after birth.

No one—regardless of race, ethnicity, sex, religion, economic level, age, or sexual orientation—is immune to STIs. Having one type of infection doesn't prevent you from acquiring another. In fact, people with STIs are *more* likely to contract the human immunodeficiency virus (HIV, the cause of AIDS) if exposed than people who don't have STIs.[9] If you had an STI in the past, this doesn't make you immune from becoming infected with it again.

There are a lot of STIs out there. Most teens have heard about syphilis and gonorrhea, which have been around for a long time; about HIV, which will kill you; about chlamydia, the most commonly reported infectious disease in the United States; and about herpes, which can permanently affect your sexual behavior. But a host of lesser-known infections can inflict varying degrees of damage.

JUST THE FACTS

STIs are more prevalent among teens than among adults. About one-fourth of all new cases occur among fifteen- to nineteen-year-olds. One out of five teens knows someone with an STI. Yet many teens underestimate their own risk for becoming infected, thinking it can't happen to them. And only a third of sexually active teens have ever been tested.[10]

STIs come in two basic varieties: bacterial and viral. The bacterial infections, such as syphilis, gonorrhea, and chlamydia, can be treated and cured with antibiotics. That's the good news. The bad news is that the amount of antibiotics needed to kill the bacteria has been escalating. Some STIs have developed resistance to antibiotics traditionally used to treat them.

The viral infections have no cure. If your teen gets a viral infection such as herpes, human papillomavirus (HPV), or HIV, she'll have it for life. Doctors can treat the symptoms, but currently they can't kill the virus without killing the body cells it's in, and we need those cells to live.

Some STIs produce symptoms that can serve as clues that your teen has become infected and needs treatment. The most common symptoms are itching, burning, and pain when urinating. Other signs like sores, blisters, or rashes, even if they go away by themselves, can also be clues.

A large percentage of women (and a small percentage of men) don't develop any symptoms. They can be infected and pass the infection on to others without knowing it. Some STIs can spread into the uterus and the fallopian tubes to cause pelvic inflammatory disease (PID), a major cause of infertility. To minimize the damage an infection can do, people who are sexually active should be checked periodically by a physician or clinic specializing in STIs, even if no symptoms are present.

So the information you need to give your teen is twofold: First, if she's sexually active, she always needs to protect herself by using a dental dam or a latex condom, preferably lubricated with a spermicide. Second, she needs to know how and where to get checked and tested periodically.

Anyone who has ever had unprotected sex should be tested for STIs. Any private physician can do the testing, but public health clinics are usually less expensive and very experienced in this field. Women should not assume that if they have a yearly checkup and Pap smear, they're okay. Most gynecologists do not routinely test for STIs.

Remind your teen that sexual responsibility is a vital ingredient in any happy, healthy sexual relationship. Encourage her to talk with her partner and exchange sexual histories, including any act of unprotected sex—vaginal, oral, or anal intercourse. If either partner in an ongoing relationship tests positive for an STI, both need to be treated, or they may keep reinfecting each other.

The old saying, "A picture is worth a thousand words," may be especially true here. You may want to show your teen pictures of genitals infected with syphilis, gonorrhea, herpes, and HPV. You can find them in books from your local library or health department. The goal is not to scare your teen, but to educate her about what these infections look like. When she decides to become sexually active, she should look at her partner's genitals for any warts, rashes, blisters, discharge, or other sores.

CENTERS FOR DISEASE CONTROL (CDC) NATIONAL STD HOTLINE

1-800-227-8922
or 1-800-342-2437

A service of the CDC's National Center for HIV, STD, and TB Prevention, Division of Sexually Transmitted Diseases, the National STD Hotline provides anonymous, confidential information on sexually transmitted diseases (STDs) and how to prevent them. It also provides referrals to clinical and other services. Operates 24 hours a day, 7 days a week. For more information, visit the Web site at *www.cdc.gov/nchstp/dstd/dstdp.html.*

Curable STIs

Most of the curable STIs are caused by bacteria. All are treatable. Often, the early symptoms are mild or unnoticeable. If they aren't treated early and effectively, these infections can spread throughout the body. Some increase the risk of acquiring and transmitting HIV.

SYPHILIS

Syphilis is one of the oldest STIs around. It is also on the decline. In the United States, syphilis rates are now at an all-time low, and it appears as though we might be able to eliminate this disease, which once caused horrible epidemics.[11] Even so, your teen should know about syphilis.

If left untreated, syphilis goes through three stages. In primary (first stage) syphilis, a painless sore appears. This sore, called a chancre (SHANK-er), has a raised rim and a hollow center. It is highly infectious.

The chancre is most often found on the part of the body that came in contact with the partner's sore during vaginal, oral, or anal intercourse. On men, that's usually the penis, where it's noticeable. On women, the chancre can be in the vagina, where it might go unnoticed. The chancre can also appear on the vulva, on the anus, in the rectum, on the lips, and in the mouth.

Most women with first-stage syphilis learn about their infection by being tested, being told by their partner—or being informed by the health department. Syphilis is a reportable disease, which means that if you test positive for it, your physician or health care professional is required by law to report it.

Whether it's treated or not, the chancre goes away after a few weeks. That doesn't mean the disease goes away. Secondary (second stage) syphilis usually starts with a highly infectious skin rash that can appear on the palms of the hands and soles of the feet, or all over the body. It usually doesn't itch. Some people will have other symptoms during this stage, such as fevers, swollen lymph glands, nausea, and loss of hair and appetite. Left untreated, the symptoms will disappear, but the disease will not.

For some people with syphilis, the disease may lapse into a latent (hidden) stage, during which there are no symptoms and the person is no longer contagious—although the disease can spread from a woman to her child during pregnancy. Without treatment, syphilis remains in the body and may begin to damage the internal organs. The internal damage may show up many years later in tertiary (third stage) syphilis. Complications of this final stage include mental illness, paralysis, blindness, heart disease, and death.

Syphilis can be diagnosed, treated, and cured at all stages with the proper dose of antibiotics (usually penicillin). The disease will be cured, but the damage already done to any body organs will not be reversed. If you have syphilis and get cured, this doesn't protect you from getting it again. If you're already on antibiotics for some other reason, this won't protect you from getting syphilis if you have unprotected sex with an infectious partner. Curing syphilis requires much larger doses of antibiotics than are usually prescribed for other conditions.

GONORRHEA

Gonorrhea is another reportable STI, although many cases go unreported. About 400,000 new cases of gonorrhea are reported to the U.S. Centers for Disease Control and Prevention (CDC) each year.[12] It's estimated that if all new cases were reported, that number would rise to somewhere between 650,000 and one million a year.[13]

Gonorrhea bacteria grow in the warm, moist mucous membranes of the body—the genital tract, mouth, rectum, and urethra. In women, the cervix is usually the first place of infection.

Gonorrhea is sometimes called the drip or the clap. In men, it causes a pus-like discharge from the penis and a burning sensation when urinating. It can also cause painful or swollen testicles. These symptoms will usually bring a man to a health care professional, where he will be tested. Some women have a yellow or bloody vaginal discharge and pain when urinating. These symptoms are easily mistaken for a bladder or vaginal infection, so the woman may or may not seek appropriate medical treatment.

Most women and some men have no symptoms at all. The only way they know if they have the disease is if they are tested. Meanwhile, once they are infected, they can spread gonorrhea to others through unprotected vaginal, oral, or anal intercourse.

Untreated gonorrhea can cause serious and permanent problems in both men and women. In women, it can spread into the uterus and the fallopian tubes, causing PID. In men, it can cause epididymitis (a painful inflammation of the epididymis, the storage area for sperm located on top of each testicle), affect the prostate, and scar the inside of the urethra. Both women and men can be made infertile. Gonorrhea can also spread to the eyes, blood, joints, heart valves, and brain. Persons with gonorrhea can more easily contract HIV.

JUST THE FACTS

In 1995, young people ages fifteen to nineteen had the highest rates of gonorrhea infection of any age group in the United States. The rates were especially high for African American teens.[14]

CHLAMYDIA

In 1999, 659,441 cases of chlamydia were reported to the CDC.[15] Meanwhile, the CDC estimates that more than three million people in the United States are infected with chlamydia each year.[16]

Why the huge gap between reported cases and estimates? Because chlamydia is a "silent" disease. It usually causes no symptoms, or the symptoms are so mild that the disease is often not diagnosed or treated until complications develop. As many as 75 percent of women and 50 percent of men with chlamydia don't know they have it and don't seek treatment for it.[17] Meanwhile, they continue to infect their partners.

Chlamydia is the most common STI in the United States today.[18] It is a special problem for teens. In some communities, studies have found that up to 30 percent of sexually active teenage women and 10 percent of sexually active teenage men are affected.[19] About half of all new chlamydia cases each year occur in girls ages fifteen to nineteen. In 1998, researchers from Johns Hopkins University suggested that all sexually active teenage girls be routinely screened for chlamydia every six months.[20]

The symptoms of chlamydia, when they exist, include an abnormal discharge from the vagina or penis, or pain while urinating. Left untreated, the disease can spread, causing PID in women and epididymitis in men. Up to 40 percent of women with untreated chlamydia develop PID.[21] Chlamydia often co-exists with gonorrhea; people may be infected with both at the same time. Women with chlamydia may also have a higher risk of acquiring HIV from an infected partner.

Many doctors now recommend that anyone who has more than one sex partner be regularly tested for chlamydia, even if they have no symptoms. The disease can be easily treated and cured with antibiotics.

When you talk with your teen about STIs, be sure to emphasize that many have no symptoms. If your teen is sexually active, he should be tested for STIs. And if he ever notices anything "strange" in his genital area—burning or discharge during urination, an unusual sore, a rash, itching, tenderness, pain—he should stop having sex and see a health care provider right away. If he has oral sex, he should know that STIs can infect the throat as well. Of course, girls should be told this, too.

PELVIC INFLAMMATORY DISEASE (PID)

According to the CDC, PID is the most common and serious complication of STIs among women, aside from AIDS. Each year in the United States, more than one million women have an episode of acute PID. The rate of infection is highest among teenagers.[22]

PID is caused by bacteria moving upward from a woman's urethra, vagina, or cervix into the upper genital tract and the internal reproductive organs, where it can scar the fallopian tubes. Most cases of PID are associated with gonorrhea and chlamydia. It is estimated that 10 to 80 percent of women with either of these STIs will develop PID.[23]

Especially when PID is caused by chlamydia, a woman may have mild symptoms or no symptoms, even as the disease is damaging her reproductive organs. The most common symptom is lower abdominal pain. Some women have a foul-smelling vaginal discharge, fever, pain during urination, pain during sexual intercourse, and/or irregular menstrual bleeding.

Left untreated, PID can lead to abscesses, chronic pelvic pain, infertility, and ectopic (tubal) pregnancy, a life-threatening condition in which a fertilized egg grows outside the uterus, usually in a fallopian tube. Ectopic pregnancy results in miscarriage and is potentially fatal for the mother.

PID can be hard to diagnose, but early and complete treatment can help prevent complications. Treatment can't reverse any damage that has already been done to the reproductive organs.

Women who douche have a higher risk of developing PID than women who don't.[24] Douching may push bacteria into the upper genital tract. It may also ease any discharge caused by an infection, so a woman might think she doesn't have to see a doctor. Tell your teen that she doesn't need to douche. All she needs to do is wash the outside of her vulva daily with a mild soap. That way, if she ever does develop an STI, douching won't hide the symptoms.

JUST the FACTS

■ More than 100,000 women become infertile each year as a result of PID.[25]

■ A large proportion of the 70,000 ectopic pregnancies that occur each year are due to the consequences of PID.[26]

■ As many as one-third of women who have had PID will have the disease at least one more time.[27]

■ More than 150 women die every year from PID.[28]

CHANCROID

Chancroid is a bacterial infection that is spread by sexual contact. In men, symptoms include painful open sores on the genitals, and sometimes swollen lymph nodes in the groin. In women, symptoms may include painful urination or defecation, painful intercourse, rectal bleeding, or vaginal discharge.

It may be difficult for some people to distinguish chancroid lesions from other sores caused by syphilis or genital herpes, so anyone with genital sores should see a doctor immediately. The disease is treatable with antibiotics. Chancroid may be associated with increased risk of transmitting HIV.

NONGONOCOCCAL URETHRITIS (NGU)

Nongonococcal urethritis (NGU) is also known as nonspecific urethritis (NSU). It is any inflammation of the urethra not caused by gonorrhea. The most common villain is chlamydia, but NGU can also be caused by other bacteria, by parasites, by fungi, or even by allergic reactions to vaginal secretions, soaps, or vaginal contraceptives.

Common symptoms are burning or tingling during urination that is sometimes accompanied by a slight (usually clear) discharge from the urethra. These symptoms appear most often in men; women rarely have any symptoms. In fact, NGU is mostly a men's disease, since the female urethra is seldom infected during intercourse.

Left untreated, NGU can lead to epididymitis in men and infection of the prostate gland. In women, it may result in cervical inflammation or PID. NGU is treated with antibiotics such as tetracycline.

BACTERIAL VAGINOSIS (BV)

Bacterial vaginosis (BV) is the most common vaginal infection in women. No one really knows what causes it, but women who have a new sex partner or who have had many partners are more likely to get it.

BV is linked to changes in the bacteria found in a woman's vagina. Normally, the vagina contains mostly "good" bacteria and fewer "harmful" bacteria. Changing the pH of the vagina (how alkaline or acidic it is) by taking antibiotics, douching, or even by taking birth control pills can sometimes lead to BV.

Symptoms include a foul-smelling, thin vaginal discharge that is white or gray. Some women may also have burning during urination, itching around the outside of the vagina, or both. Some women have no symptoms at all.

In most cases, BV has no complications. But it sometimes leads to PID, and it can make a woman more susceptible to other STIs including gonorrhea, chlamydia, and HIV. In some cases, BV clears up on its own without treatment. Waiting for that to happen is never a good idea. Any abnormal symptoms or conditions should always be checked out by a health care professional.

Men whose partners have BV should be checked and treated, even though the men probably won't have symptoms. This will prevent the infection from ping-ponging back and forth between the partners.

TRICHOMONIASIS

Trichomoniasis, also called trich, is an infection caused by a microscopic single-celled protozoan parasite. The parasite can live in a woman's vagina and vulva or a man's urethra.

The most common symptom of trichomoniasis in women is a frothy, yellow-green vaginal discharge with an unpleasant smell, which can cause the vulva to become irritated, itchy, and sore. Women may also experience painful urination and lower abdominal pain. Frequently, there are no symptoms. Men almost never have symptoms, but some might have a thin, whitish discharge from the penis and painful or difficult urination.

When one partner is diagnosed with trichomoniasis, both partners should be treated to eliminate the parasite. It's uncommon, though possible, for the organism to invade the urethra and bladder. Left untreated, it can damage the cells of the cervix. Trichomoniasis may be associated with increased risk of transmitting HIV.

VAGINAL YEAST INFECTION

Doctors estimate that about 75 percent of all women will have at least one symptomatic yeast infection during their lifetimes.[29] Vaginal yeast infections are an overgrowth of a fungus that lives in a healthy vagina, usually without causing any problems.

Overgrowth can happen for many reasons. Antibiotics, birth control pills, douching, perfumed feminine hygiene sprays, and a change in diet can all upset the vagina's natural balance. Diabetes raises blood sugar levels, and yeast love a sugary environment. Uncontrolled diabetes may result in more yeast infections.

Even wearing tight, poorly ventilated clothing and underwear, or wearing a damp bathing suit or pantyhose for hours, can increase a woman's chance of getting a yeast infection, since yeast thrive in warmth and humidity. It is not known for sure if yeast can be transmitted sexually, but it's probably best not to have sexual intercourse when a yeast infection is present.

The most common symptoms of yeast infection in women are itching, burning, and irritation of the vagina and vulva. Some women have a white, clumpy discharge that looks like cottage cheese. Other women have a watery discharge or none. Most male partners of women with vaginal yeast infection don't have any symptoms. Some men may have an itchy rash or burning sensation after unprotected intercourse.

Medications that treat yeast infections are available over the counter. Before using any of them, your teen should see a doctor. She may have a vaginal yeast infection—or she may have BV, trichomoniasis, or an STI. Your teen won't be able to tell, but a doctor will.

PUBIC LICE

Pubic lice, commonly called crabs, are very tiny insects that survive by feeding on human blood. They have claws that help them to hold onto hair, most commonly pubic hair. They bite into skin and cause intense itching. They lay eggs, called nits, which can fall off the pubic hair and onto clothing, towels, bed sheets, etc., where they can be passed on to others. You can actually see both the whitish eggs and the lice themselves, if you look very carefully.

If your teen gets pubic lice, there are creams, lotions, and shampoos available that will kill the lice and its eggs. All of her clothing and bed linens will need to be dry-cleaned or washed in very hot water (125° F), dried at a high setting, and ironed if possible.

Pubic lice are most often spread by sexual contact. In some cases, they can be picked up from someone else's infested clothing or bedding. To be on the safe side, anyone your teen has come into close contact with—including family and close friends—should also be treated.

The lice die within 24 hours of being separated from the body, but the eggs may live for up to six days, so any treatment should be applied for the full time recommended.

SCABIES

Like pubic lice, scabies—tiny mites—are spread primarily through sexual contact. They are also transmitted by contact with skin, infested clothing, sheets, or towels, and even furniture. Scabies are highly contagious.

The female mite burrows into the skin—usually on the hands (between the fingers), wrists, elbows, lower abdomen, and genitals—to lay her eggs. Small red bumps or lines appear and cause intense itching. The skin reaction might not happen until a month or even longer after infestation. During this time, a person may pass the disease to a sex partner or anyone else he comes into close contact with.

Scabies may be confused with poison ivy or eczema, so anyone with these symptoms should see a health care professional for an accurate diagnosis and effective treatment. Family members, close friends, and sex partners should also be treated. Clothing, bedding, towels, and furniture should be cleaned.

Incurable STIs

Chlamydia, gonorrhea, chancroid, crabs—nobody wants any of these STIs. But at least they can all be treated and cured. For the viral STIs, some of the symptoms can be treated, but cures for the diseases have not yet been found. If your teen acquires a viral STI, she will probably have it for the rest of her life. She needs to know how serious these STIs are.

HERPES

Somewhere around 45 million Americans already have genital herpes. About one million more will get it this year.[30] These estimates are probably conservative, since doctors aren't required to report herpes.

Herpes is caused by the herpes simplex virus (HSV), part of a family of viruses that also cause chicken pox, shingles, and mononucleosis (mono). There are two types of HSV. Type 1 (HSV-1) causes oral herpes (fever blisters and cold sores on the mouth), but it can also infect the genitals during oral sex. Type 2 (HSV-2) is the usual cause of genital herpes, but it can also infect the mouth during oral sex.

Both types can cause painful fluid-filled blisters that are packed with viral material and are highly contagious. Sores can also appear on the buttocks or thighs, in the urinary tract, inside a woman's vagina or on her cervix, and on other parts of the body where the virus has entered through broken skin.

Herpes is spread by skin-to-skin contact with a contagious area—which may be a blister, but can also include skin that does not appear to be broken or have a sore. The virus likes moist areas of the body, which is why the mouth, genitals, and anal areas are such good hosts. A person who touches a cold sore on his own mouth, then touches his genitals or anus without first washing his hands with soap and water, can spread the infection to a new area on his body.

There are no documented cases of a person getting genital herpes from an inanimate object such as a toilet seat, bathtub, or towel. Herpes is a very fragile virus and does not live long on surfaces.[31]

Different people have different symptoms. Some people might have an itching, burning, or tingling feeling in the genital or anal area, or any area where a blister is about to form. Some might have a fever, headache, or muscle aches; pain in the legs, buttocks, or genital area; a vaginal or penile discharge; painful or difficult urination; swollen glands in the groin area; or a feeling of pressure in the abdomen. A person may show symptoms within days after getting infected—or it may take weeks, months, or years. Some people never have any symptoms, but they can still spread the disease.

Your teen may be surprised to learn that cold sores, fever blisters, and stress blisters are caused by herpes. ("I just have a cold sore. I don't have herpes!") About 50 to 80 percent of the adult population in the United States has oral herpes.[32] Most people are infected as children, when they are kissed by a friend or a relative. Sexual contact isn't necessary to spread the Type 1 virus. The blisters will go away after one to three weeks, but the virus never does.

Some people who contract herpes only have one outbreak. Others have frequent outbreaks. While doctors don't quite understand this, we do know that some things—illness, poor diet, stress—can trigger a herpes outbreak, which usually occurs at the site of the first infection. We had a young client who had an outbreak every month when she began to menstruate.

Although herpes can't be cured, some antiviral medications can cut back the frequency and severity of the outbreaks. They can help speed the healing process. Living a healthier life—eating well, getting enough exercise and sleep, managing stress—can help reduce the frequency of outbreaks.

Women with genital herpes are at greater risk for cervical cancer, which is the second most common form of cancer in women.[33] If a woman has an outbreak while she is pregnant, she can pass the virus to her unborn child. Half of the babies infected with herpes either die or suffer from nerve damage.[34] If a woman is having an outbreak during labor and delivery, her doctor will usually do a Cesarean section to protect the baby.

Men and women with herpes risk transferring the virus to their eyes, causing a potentially serious eye infection known as ocular herpes, or herpes keratitis. If your teen gets cold sores, warn her to leave them alone. If she touches them, she should wash her hands with soap and water immediately after.

Anyone who is about to have oral, genital, or anal contact should look carefully at what they are about to touch, kiss, or fondle. If there is a sore, they should think again. If your teen has a sore, suggest that she refrain from kissing lips—or anything else. While herpes isn't fatal, it is an unpleasant house guest that stays for life.

NATIONAL HERPES HOTLINE

(919) 361-8488

The National Herpes Hotline is operated by the American Social Health Association (ASHA) as part of the Herpes Resource Center (HRC). The hotline provides accurate information and appropriate referrals to anyone concerned about herpes. Trained Health Communication Specialists are available to address questions related to transmission, prevention, and treatment. The hotline also provides support for emotional issues surrounding herpes, such as self-esteem and partner communication. Hours: 9 A.M. to 6 P.M., EST, Monday through Friday. For more information, visit the Web site at *www.ashastd.org/hrc/index.html.*

HUMAN PAPILLOMAVIRUS (HPV)

You've probably heard human papillomavirus (HPV) called by a different name—genital warts or venereal warts. In fact, HPV is a family of more than one hundred viruses. Some types cause genital warts, and some cause no noticeable symptoms. Other types of HPV can lead to cervical, penile, and anal cancer. A recent study has linked HPV with oral cancer, and there is some evidence showing that oral HPV is acquired through oral sex.[35] So oral sex isn't as safe as some teens might think.

JUST THE FACTS

■ HPV is so common that most of the world's sexually active people may be infected with it.[36]

■ An estimated 5.5 million people become infected with HPV each year in the United States. An estimated 20 million Americans are currently infected.[37]

■ Studies repeatedly show high levels of HPV infection in women, with the highest levels among young women.[38]

Thirty types of HPV can infect the genital area, and it is some of these that cause genital warts. The warts can be soft, pinkish lesions (usually in moist areas like the vulva, vagina, anus, or urethra) or harder, grayish-white bumps (in drier areas like the shaft of the penis). The warts may cause itching or burning around the genitals; they may not. The warts are very contagious and are spread through oral, genital, or anal sex with an infected partner. They can also be spread by touching or rubbing an infected area.

Genital warts often disappear without treatment. When they don't, various treatment options are available. The warts can be frozen, cauterized, surgically removed, or treated with creams and solutions. Over-the-counter wart treatments should *never* be used in the genital area. Although there is currently no "cure" for genital HPV infection (or any other viral STI), most cases are transient. They clear themselves through the natural immune process, without medical intervention.

If a woman has an abnormal Pap smear, this may indicate a precancerous condition of the cervix that is caused by HPV. Medical follow-up and treatment can help ensure that infected cells don't develop into cervical cancer.

Because HPV is so widespread and there are so many strains of the virus, the only way to avoid it is to never have sexual contact with anyone. Two uninfected people who have never had any other partners besides each other can't get genital HPV. Correct and consistent use of condoms can reduce but not eliminate—the risk of getting or transmitting HPV. The virus can often be found on the dry skin surrounding the groin and stomach—areas a condom doesn't cover.

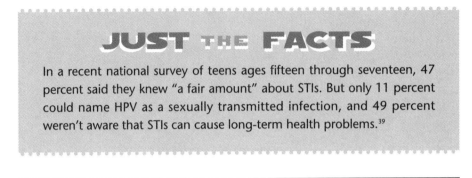

JUST THE FACTS

In a recent national survey of teens ages fifteen through seventeen, 47 percent said they knew "a fair amount" about STIs. But only 11 percent could name HPV as a sexually transmitted infection, and 49 percent weren't aware that STIs can cause long-term health problems.[39]

NATIONAL HPV AND CERVICAL CANCER PREVENTION HOTLINE

(919) 361-4848

The National HPV and Cervical Cancer Prevention Hotline is operated by the American Social Health Association (ASHA) as part of the HPV and Cervical Cancer Prevention Resource Center. It provides current information on the virus and its link to cancer through free information to the public about risk reduction, diagnosis, and treatment of HPV and the prevention of cervical cancer, including the most up-to-date FDA-approved technologies. Trained Health Communication Specialists are available to address questions related to transmission, prevention, and treatment of HPV. The hotline also provides support for emotional issues surrounding HPV, such as self-esteem and partner communication. Hours: 1 P.M. to 6 P.M., EST, Monday through Friday. For more information, visit the Web site at *www.ashastd.org/hpvccrc/index.html*.

HEPATITIS B VIRUS (HBV)

There are five types of hepatitis virus—A, B, C, D, and E—all of which attack the liver. Hepatitis A can be spread by sexual contact (usually when the mouth comes in contact with something that has been contaminated with the stool of a person with hepatitis A), but the hepatitis B virus (HBV) is the one most closely associated with sexual transmission, and the one that can result in chronic infection. A vaccine that prevents HBV has been available since 1981 (and a hepatitis A vaccine has been available since 1995), but many teens and young adults have not been vaccinated.

Many people infected with HBV don't have any symptoms at all. Some people have mild flu-like symptoms (achiness, nausea) that just won't go away. Other possible symptoms include severe fatigue, loss of appetite, abdominal tenderness, vomiting, and jaundice (yellowing of the skin and the whites of the eyes).

HBV is highly contagious. It is spread by having vaginal, oral, or anal intercourse with an infected person, sharing personal items with infected blood on them (such as toothbrushes and razors), and using contaminated needles. People who have sex with more than one partner are at high risk. So are drug users, men who have sex with men, health care workers—and people who get tattoos or piercings. Babies born to infected mothers should be vaccinated within twelve hours of birth.

JUST THE FACTS

■ Hepatitis A and hepatitis B are the only STIs that are preventable with vaccination.[40]

■ About 80,000 unvaccinated people in the United States contracted hepatitis B in 1999.[41]

Antiviral drugs may relieve some symptoms and reduce an infected person's chance of getting severe liver disease. Rest and drinking lots of fluids are usually recommended. Some people's immune system fights off the infection. Other people stay infected for life and can spread the disease. Lifelong infection increases the chances that the person will get cirrhosis (scarring) of the liver or liver cancer. Each year, 5,000 people in the United States die from liver disease caused by HBV.[42]

The CDC recommends that everyone under nineteen years old be vaccinated against HBV. The vaccine is safe and effective. After you complete the three-shot series, you don't need booster shots. If your teen hasn't been vaccinated, talk with your teen and your family doctor. Arrange for your teen to be vaccinated.

HEPATITIS HOTLINE

1-888-4-HEP-CDC
(1-888-443-7232)

A service of the CDC's Division of Viral Hepatitis, this 24-hour hot-line provides recorded information and fact sheets by fax. There is also an option to speak to a live counselor about viral hepatitis issues. For more information, visit the Web site at *www.cdc.gov/ncidod/diseases/hepatitis/index.htm.*

HUMAN IMMUNODEFICIENCY VIRUS (HIV)

On July 27, 1982, federal officials, university researchers, community activists, and others met in Washington, D.C., and named a mysterious new disease: AIDS, for Acquired Immuno Deficiency Syndrome. At that time, the CDC had reported 413 cases of the disease in the United States, with 155 deaths.

By the end of the year 2000, nearly 22 million people worldwide had died from HIV/AIDS. An estimated 36.1 million people were living with HIV/AIDS. About 15,000 more people were being infected every day.[43] What started as a mystery had become a global epidemic and the most serious and devastating of all viral STIs.

When AIDS was first noted in the United States, the highest rates of infection were among gay men and intravenous (IV) drug users. Education efforts in the gay community led to a decline in infection rates among older gay men. Today, HIV-related illness and death have the greatest impact on young people.

JUST the FACTS

■ Approximately 40,000 new HIV infections occur each year in the United States, about 70 percent among men and 30 percent among women. Of these newly infected people, half are younger than twenty-five years of age,[44] and one-quarter are under twenty-one.[45]

■ Between 1990 and 1995, AIDS incidence among young gay and bisexual men and IV drug users stayed relatively constant, but it rose more than 130 percent among young heterosexual men and women.[46]

AIDS is caused by the human immunodeficiency virus (HIV). This virus attacks the body's immune system and, over time, leaves the infected person unable to fight off disease. People with AIDS are susceptible to many life-threatening diseases (opportunistic infections) and to certain forms of cancer.

Testing positive for HIV is very different from having AIDS. A person isn't diagnosed with AIDS until the HIV virus reaches a certain concentration in the blood. A person who has been infected with HIV will test positive within three to six months of exposure to the virus. Anyone who has an act of unprotected sex should be tested, start using (or go back to using) latex condoms consistently and correctly, and get tested again in six months.

HIV is spread through the exchange of vaginal secretions, semen, blood, breast milk, and other body fluids containing blood. Just one contact with an infected body fluid can result in infection. You can't, however, get HIV through casual contact, such as sharing a soda, hugging a friend, shaking hands, social kissing, or sitting on a toilet seat. You can't get it from mosquitoes who have bitten people with HIV.

You get HIV by having sexual contact (vaginal, oral, or anal) with an infected person, by sharing needles or syringes with someone who is infected, or (more rarely now that blood is screened) through transfusions of infected blood or blood clotting factors. Babies born to HIV-infected women may become infected before or during birth, or through breast-feeding after birth. Having STIs other than AIDS increases your risk for becoming infected with HIV.

Some people with HIV/AIDS are able to take expensive "drug cocktails" that slow the progress of the disease. They are living longer and healthier lives. But no cure or vaccine yet exists for the virus. At this time, it is still almost always fatal.

The symptoms of HIV infection are many and varied: fatigue, fever, cough, weight loss, headache, diarrhea, seizures, infections. Because the symptoms remind people of other diseases, they may not seek medical care. Many people carry the HIV virus for as long as ten years (maybe longer) without developing any symptoms. Meanwhile, they pass the virus on to others. The CDC estimates that as many as one in three people with HIV don't know they have it.[47]

The CDC is especially concerned about improving HIV prevention for young people. Research has shown that early, clear communication between parents and young people about sex is an important step in helping teens adopt and maintain safer sex behaviors.[48]

CDC NATIONAL AIDS HOTLINE

1-800-342-AIDS
(1-800-342-2437)

One of the first government services established to respond to the public's questions about the AIDS epidemic, the National AIDS Hotline is the world's largest health information service. It operates 24 hours a day, 7 days a week. Trained information specialists answer questions about HIV infection and AIDS and provide referrals to appropriate services including clinics, hospitals, local hotlines, counseling and testing sites, legal services, health departments, support groups, educational organizations, and service agencies throughout the United States. Callers can also order various publications, posters, and other informational materials from the CDC National Prevention Information Network through the Hotline. For more information, visit the Web site at *www.cdc.gov/hiv/hivinfo/nah.htm.*

History Quiz

All teens need to understand that the more sexual partners they have, the more likely they are to get an STI. When they have sexual contact with someone, they're having sexual contact with all the partners that person has ever had. Any one of those earlier partners could have been carrying an STI and passed it on without knowing it, and without showing any symptoms.

Just because someone looks great doesn't mean that he or she is free of infection. Just because someone is a member of one group or another doesn't mean that he or she is free of infection. STIs cut across all racial, religious, ethnic, and class lines.

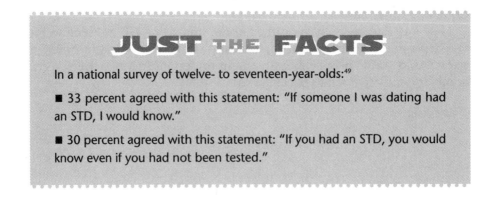

JUST THE FACTS

In a national survey of twelve- to seventeen-year-olds:[49]

■ 33 percent agreed with this statement: "If someone I was dating had an STD, I would know."

■ 30 percent agreed with this statement: "If you had an STD, you would know even if you had not been tested."

■ 22 percent agreed with this statement: "Unless you have sex with lots of partners, STDs are not something you have to worry about."

Before your teen has any type of sexual contact with another person, she should ask four specific questions about the person's sexual history:

1. "Have you ever had an act of unprotected sex?" If the answer is yes, the person might not be safe.

2. "Have you ever tested positive for a sexually transmitted infection?" If the answer is yes, the person might not be safe.

3. "When was the last time you were tested for a sexually transmitted infection?" If the answer is "longer than three months ago," the person might not be safe.

4. "Have you had an act of unprotected sex since being tested?" If the answer is yes, the person might not be safe.

Your teen should be equally honest about her own sexual history.

What if she seems reluctant to share sexual histories with a potential partner? Talk about that directly. If your teen says something like, "I could never ask that!" you might say, "I know it's hard, but it's really important, because you need that information to make a responsible decision." Or, "If you can't talk honestly with your potential partner, why would you even consider having sexual contact with [him or her]?"

Most teens (and adults) find it very difficult to initiate this kind of conversation. It may help if they start by reassuring the other person that they're not making accusations. They can also break the ice by volunteering their own sexual history first.

Honesty is the best foundation for any relationship. Knowing each other's sexual history ahead of time is essential to making a decision that could affect both of their lives—forever.

JUST THE FACTS

In a national survey of sexually experienced teens ages fifteen to seventeen:[50]

■ 55 percent said they had not discussed STDs with their current or most recent sexual partner.

■ 40 percent said they had never discussed STDs with a health care provider.

- ■ 39 percent said they would be uncomfortable discussing STDs with a sexual partner.

- ■ 70 percent agreed with the statement, "It is often more embarrassing for couples to talk about sexual issues, like STDs, than to have sex."

Reducing the Risk

Total sexual abstinence—no sexual activity of any kind with any partner—is the only 100 percent effective way for your teen to protect himself from an STI. But abstinence only works as long as it's maintained, and abstinent teens (and adults) sometimes have lapses.

For those who do engage in sexual activities, using a latex condom consistently and correctly during every sexual encounter is the next safest thing. Lubricating the condom with the spermicide nonoxynol-9 may also be helpful, since there's some evidence that it kills some infections. Nonoxynol-9 all by itself will not protect the user completely, and one study seemed to indicate that it may actually increase the chances of transmitting HIV.[51]

Even with those precautions, anyone who sees a rash, sore, bump, wart, or anything that looks unusual, especially on the genitals, should stop. What if the partner says, "That's always been there," or "Oh, that? That's nothing!" or "Don't you trust me?" Tell your teen that he should stop anyway. It's not a matter of trust—it's a matter of health. Both partners can go to a doctor or a local health department clinic together to find out what they're dealing with.

But not all STIs have visible symptoms, and not even a latex condom generously lubricated with nonoxynol-9 is an absolute guarantee against an STI. Remind your teen that there's no such thing as safe sex. Tell him to know his partners and their sexual histories, to share his own sexual history, to be very careful, and to always use safer sex practices.

Give your teen a copy of "Rate the Risk" on page 202. After he completes the exercise, talk about it together. (You'll find the answers on page 203.) Your goal is to find out how knowledgeable your teen really is when it comes to sexual activities—and to help him discover what he does and doesn't know. If you prefer, you can do the exercise out loud. Then tell your teen what you want him to do if he thinks he may have an STI. Should he talk with you? See your family doctor? Go to a community clinic? If you prefer that he go to a clinic, does he know where one is and how to get there?

Preventing STIs and Pregnancy

Just as your teen needs to know about STIs and where babies come from, she also needs to know how to prevent STIs and unwanted pregnancy. You can't assume that she'll get balanced, factual information from other sources. If you want your teen to make healthy decisions, help her by being as open and honest as you can.*

THE CONDOM

The simplest and most important way to prevent STIs and pregnancies is the humble latex condom. Latex condoms prevent body fluids, bacteria, and viruses from passing from one person to another. Simply telling your teen to use a condom is not enough. Your son—and your daughter—both need to know the proper way to select, store, put on, use, take off, and dispose of a condom.

JUST THE FACTS

■ Using a condom during intercourse is more than 10,000 times safer than not using a condom.[52]

■ Condoms are 98 percent effective in preventing pregnancy when used correctly—and up to 99.9 percent effective in reducing the risk of STI transmission when combined with spermicide.[53]

■ The first-year pregnancy failure rate among typical condom users averages about 12 percent and includes pregnancies resulting from errors in condom use.[54]

Using a condom properly requires physical as well as cognitive skills. Where is your teen going to learn these skills if you don't teach them? Most sex education programs don't even mention condoms, and if they do, they seldom explain their proper use. They almost never provide any practice. This is not something you want your teen to learn by trial and error—the stakes are too high. Teens need to practice.

The 12 percent pregnancy failure rate cited above can be reduced by using the condom and a spermicide (a chemical that kills sperm) together—and by knowing how to put on a condom and take it off. Spermicides come in the form of contraceptive foams, creams, suppositories, and films. If the condom breaks or slips off, there's still some protection against pregnancy.

Teens often worry about condom size, but latex stretches and one size fits all. (Condom manufacturers offer a large size, as well as a far less popular small size, but that's mostly a marketing strategy.) In our seminars with

---

* See also "Teen Pregnancy" on pages 98–100.

teens, we demonstrate this stretchiness by placing a condom over an entire fist, right down to the wrist and beyond.

If you're comfortable doing this demonstration, you might say something like, "Some people worry that an erect penis is too big for a regular condom. Watch this." If the condom breaks, and sometimes it does, that's a great opportunity for another lesson. You could say, "Condoms aren't perfectly safe. What just happened could happen to you during a real sexual experience. That's why you should also use a spermicide."

There's a wide variety of condoms available on the market. Which are best to use? Both the Food and Drug Administration (FDA) and the CDC recommend condoms made of latex, which are regulated in the United States and must meet FDA standards. Lubricating the condom with the spermicide nonoxynol-9 may add more protection from conception and some STIs.*

Ultra-thin condoms made of animal skin (labeled "lambskin" but usually sheep intestine) are more "natural," but animal skin, like human skin, is porous, and disease agents can penetrate it. These condoms may be used for pregnancy prevention, but not to block transmission of STIs.

Condoms made from polyurethane are more expensive but appear to be as safe as latex. The FDA has approved the marketing of polyurethane condoms for people allergic to latex. Studies are still underway to determine if polyurethane is as effective as latex in preventing pregnancy and blocking STIs.

Some condoms have a tip, or receptacle, at the end. This allows a place for the ejaculate to go safely. Flavored condoms are available specifically for protection against STIs during oral sex. Because they are not lubricated with nonoxynol-9, flavored condoms are not quite as effective in preventing pregnancy.

Ribbed condoms suggest extra pleasure for a woman, but many women say they can't feel any difference. That makes sense, since the back of the vagina is relatively insensitive. Colored condoms add variety but are otherwise the same.

Many young men keep a condom in their wallet "just in case." That may seem like a smart idea, but it's not. Neither is keeping one in a pants pocket or glove compartment. Body heat and large temperature changes can affect latex. Condoms should be stored in a cool, dry place where they're safe from punctures and temperature changes. Loose jacket pockets, protected areas of a purse or backpack, or an eyeglass case are all good. And men aren't the only ones who can carry condoms. Sexually active women should carry them, too.

Old condoms can be dry, brittle, or weakened and can break more easily. Condom packages are printed with expiration dates. Tell your teen to check the expiration date carefully before using a condom. If the date has passed, the condom should be thrown away.

---

* Condoms cannot eliminate the risk of transmitting human papillomavirus (HPV). There is some controversy about whether nonoxynol-9 increases the chances of HIV infection. See note 51 on page 226.

Some teens may worry that stopping to put a condom on will "destroy the mood." You might remind your teen that an unplanned pregnancy or an STI can destroy a lot more moods. A condom can be put on at any time during foreplay, as long as the penis is erect. In fact, it should be in place before the penis has any contact with the vagina, mouth, or anal area.

Many of the teens (and parents) we talk with have never learned the proper way to put on and take off a condom. On pages 204–205, you'll find complete instructions. Review them with your teen, and give your teen a copy. Share this information with your daughter as well as your son.

Your teen should understand and practice these steps—before the heat of the moment. There are many ways to help your teen learn to use a condom properly. Some parents demonstrate them on fruits and vegetables—cucumbers, carrots, or bananas. If you're not comfortable doing this, you might try this exercise we learned from a Planned Parenthood educator many years ago and have since expanded on.

Try This

Write each of the following statements on a 3" x 5" note card (or small piece of paper). Don't write the numbers—just the words.

(1) Get a lubricated latex condom with a receptacle tip

(2) Check the expiration date

(3) Foreplay and sexual arousal

(4) Erection

(5) Carefully open the package containing the condom

(6) Leave room at the tip of the condom (pinch an inch)

(7) Roll the condom down to the very bottom of the erect penis

(8) Sexual activity

(9) Orgasm (ejaculation)

(10) Hold the rim of the condom firmly

(11) Withdraw the penis while still erect

(12) Move the condom-covered penis away from the partner

(13) Grip the rim of the condom, expand, and remove from the penis

(14) Tie the condom or wrap it in a tissue and throw it away

(15) Wash hands with soap and water

(16) Urinate

continued ——➤

> Shuffle the cards. Give them to your teen and ask her to put them in the right order. Then check her order against the numbered list above. This exercise should provide good opportunities for conversation.

THE FEMALE CONDOM

In 1993, the FDA approved the Reality female condom. This is a polyurethane pouch that fits inside a woman's vagina. It has flexible rings at both ends. The closed end is inserted deep into the vagina, like a diaphragm, where one ring holds it in place. The ring at the open end extends outside the vaginal opening and partly covers the labia. The pouch collects semen and keeps it from entering the vagina.

Female condoms are not considered as effective as latex male condoms. A limited study of this condom as a contraceptive indicates a failure rate of about 26 percent in one year. In laboratory studies, the female condom blocked viruses (which are smaller than bacteria), but more research is needed to determine how well it prevents transmission of HIV.[55]

The male and female condom cannot be used at the same time. If used together, both products will not stay in place.

The female condom isn't ideal. Sometimes the penis can slip between the pouch and the walls of the vagina, or push the outer ring into the vagina. Partners need to make sure that the penis goes *inside* the pouch. Some women experience vaginal irritation from using the female condom. But if a man can't or won't use a condom, a female condom can help guard against pregnancy and STIs.

Tell your teen that she can buy female condoms at drugstores and some supermarkets. They do cost more than male condoms.

NONPRESCRIPTION BIRTH CONTROL

Foams, creams, jellies, films, and suppositories are just different methods of delivering spermicides into the vagina. They're inexpensive, don't require a prescription, and can be bought at most supermarkets and all drug stores by anyone at any age. No one will ask for ID.

These products are easy to use, although some people find them messy, because after a period of time they liquefy and drip out of the vagina. A tissue, a panty liner, or a bit of toilet paper near the vulva will help absorb the liquid.

Spermicides should be inserted no more than twenty minutes before intercourse. They need to be inserted deep into the vagina in order to deliver the sperm-killing agent to the tip of the uterus, or cervix. If another act of intercourse is engaged in, a second application of the spermicide must be used.

Despite the claims made on the labels, the protection spermicides offer is imperfect. Of one hundred women who use contraceptive foam, cream, jelly, film, or suppositories, twenty-six will become pregnant during the first year of typical use.[56] These failures may be the result of not following the directions correctly, inserting the spermicide too early, or not getting the applicator far enough back into the vagina to cover the cervix completely. Because of these possibilities, we recommend using two applications for each act of intercourse.

For the best protection against pregnancy, spermicides should be used in combination with a latex condom. They should not be considered effective protection against STIs.

PRESCRIPTION BIRTH CONTROL

Before a young woman chooses to be sexually active, she should visit a gynecologist for a thorough examination. If your daughter is uncomfortable with this, you may say something like, "If it bothers you too much to go to a doctor, maybe you're not ready for sexual intercourse." A health care professional can discuss the birth control options available and help her choose what's best for her.

Some of these choices—including diaphragms, intrauterine devices (IUDs), cervical caps, birth control pills, Norplant, Depo-Provera ("depo") shots, Lunelle (a new monthly shot), and the new vaginal contraceptive ring (approved by the FDA in October 2001)—are only available by prescription. A gynecologist or an organization such as Planned Parenthood will give your teen specific instructions on how these work. Encourage your teen to ask questions about anything she doesn't understand. Make sure she knows that no form of prescription birth control will protect her against STIs.

You should also encourage your son to become knowledgeable about all the different forms of birth control. Tell him that a supportive, informed partner is a vital component of a healthy relationship.

JUST the FACTS

In a recent national survey of teens ages fifteen through seventeen:[57]

■ 21 percent said that birth control pills are effective in preventing HIV.

■ 22 percent said that birth control pills are effective in preventing other STDs.

NATURAL BIRTH CONTROL

Natural birth control—sometimes called the rhythm method—involves using a calendar and body clues (like temperature and vaginal secretions) to determine when a woman is ovulating and therefore fertile. The couple attempts to time intercourse in such a way that live sperm won't be in the woman's body just before, during, or after ovulation. Some people use this method because their religion does not condone other forms of birth control.

These natural clues may not be easy to detect, and many things can throw a woman's menstrual cycle out of kilter. If she's under stress, catches a cold, gets the flu, or simply is worried about getting pregnant, her cycle can change. It's also common for young women's menstrual cycles to be somewhat irregular for the first several years, which may make determining ovulation even more difficult.

Another problem with the rhythm method is that sperm can live inside a woman's body for at least seventy-two hours, and sometimes longer. If a woman has intercourse on what she believes is a safe day and then ovulates unexpectedly a day or two later, she can still get pregnant. And, of course, this method provides no protection against STIs.

Still, if abstinence and other methods of birth control are not an option, the rhythm method is better than nothing. It is best practiced within a monogamous long-term relationship. It takes months of training, careful record-keeping, and the willingness of both partners to avoid taking risks during "unsafe" days.

WITHDRAWAL

Some teens think that coitus interruptus—also known as withdrawal, or pulling the penis out of the vagina before ejaculation—is a form of birth control. In fact, it doesn't work well, and it provides no protection against STIs.

First, there's the obvious risk that, even with the best intentions, the man may not be able to control when he ejaculates. Second, even if the man ejaculates near the opening of the vagina, not in it, pregnancy is still a possibility. Sperm deposited on the inner thigh of a woman, or anywhere near the vaginal opening, can make their way inside. Third, a man doesn't have to ejaculate to cause a pregnancy. The pre-ejaculatory fluid secreted by the Cowper's gland to neutralize the acid in the urethra may contain some sperm.

For all of these reasons (and maybe more), withdrawal is not a safe option. Talk with your teen about the many risks of withdrawal.

YOU CAN'T GET PREGNANT IF . . . MYTHS

Many teens believe all kinds of myths about birth control. Since most teens are smart about lots of other things, it's hard to imagine that they can be so easily fooled about something so important. But they can be, and they often are, and the results can be serious and life-changing.

TRUE OR FALSE?

Read the following statements aloud to your teen. For each, she should respond "True" or "False." If your teen is a boy, simply rephrase the questions. ("You can't a girl pregnant if it's her first time." "You can't get a girl pregnant if you pull out before you ejaculate, or if you don't go all the way in.") **All statements are false.** If you discover that your teen believes one or more of the myths, take this opportunity to tell her about effective birth control methods including abstinence, condoms, and birth control pills.

- You can't get pregnant if it's your first time.
- You can't get pregnant if you're both virgins.
- You can't get pregnant if you're having your period.
- You can't get pregnant if the guy pulls out before he ejaculates, or if he doesn't go all the way in.
- You can't get pregnant if you have sexual intercourse standing up.
- You can't get pregnant if you have sex in a pool or a hot tub.
- You can't get pregnant if you douche with a cola soft drink after sex.
- You can't get pregnant if you douche with vinegar after sex.
- You can't get pregnant if you don't have an orgasm.
- You can't get pregnant if you and your partner don't experience orgasm at the same time.
- You can't get pregnant if you jump up and down after sexual intercourse (to get all the sperm out).
- You can't get pregnant if you push really hard on your belly button after sexual intercourse.
- You can't get pregnant if you take a shower or bath right after sexual intercourse.
- You can't get pregnant if you're on top during sexual intercourse.
- You can't get pregnant if you take aspirin and drink a cola soft drink after sexual intercourse.
- You can't get pregnant if you make yourself sneeze for fifteen minutes after sexual intercourse.

continued ⟶

Adapted from "Fact Sheet: You Can't Get Pregnant If You Do It Standing Up . . . and Other Myths," National Campaign to Prevent Teen Pregnancy, April 2000; *www.teenpregnancy.org*, (202) 478-8500. Used with permission.

You might also check out your teen's opinions on other myths about contraception and sexual health:

- It's okay to use your friend's or sister's birth control pills.
- You only take birth control pills when you're going to have sexual intercourse.
- People can't get sexually transmitted infections from having oral sex.
- Other people can tell if you're a virgin by looking at you.
- Other people can tell if you have a sexually transmitted infection by looking at you.
- If you stop having sex with a guy once he's aroused, he will be in serious pain.

Adapted from "Fact Sheet: You Can't Get Pregnant If You Do It Standing Up . . . and Other Myths," National Campaign to Prevent Teen Pregnancy, April 2000; *www.teenpregnancy.org,* (202) 478-8500. Used with permission.

EMERGENCY CONTRACEPTION (EC)

What if a condom breaks, or an act of unprotected sexual intercourse takes place? Few teens know about emergency contraception (EC) options that can help prevent an unwanted pregnancy. If you want your teen to be fully informed, tell her about the choices available today. Tell her your views and listen to hers.

Many people believe that EC causes an abortion. In fact, according to medical science, it prevents a pregnancy from happening, which makes abortion unnecessary. Medical science defines the beginning of pregnancy as the implantation of the fertilized egg in the lining of a woman's uterus, which begins five to seven days after fertilization and ends several days later. EC prevents implantation. If the fertilized egg has already implanted, EC won't work. EC has been available for more than 25 years and could prevent 1.7 million unintended pregnancies and 800,000 abortions each year.[58]

Currently there are two main types of EC. Both require a prescription in most states, and neither provides protection against STIs. They are called "emergency contraception" because they should only be used in emergencies—as a backup, not as regular birth control.

Emergency contraceptive pills (ECPs) contain hormones that are used in some kinds of ordinary birth control pills. They are often called "morning after pills," but this is misleading for two reasons. First, the pills are taken in two doses, not just one. Second, they don't have to be taken the morning after unprotected intercourse. The first dose should be taken within seventy-two hours (three days) of unprotected intercourse, and the second dose twelve hours later.[59] The sooner ECPs are taken after unprotected intercourse, the more effective they are.[60]

Almost every woman who needs EC can safely use ECPs.[61] Some women experience side effects—nausea, vomiting, breast tenderness, fatigue, headaches, irregular bleeding, abdominal pain—that usually disappear one or two days after the second dose. If a woman is already pregnant, the ECPs won't work.

The second type of EC involves inserting a copper-releasing IUD into the woman's uterus. This can be done within five days of unprotected intercourse.[62] A woman should not use this form of EC if she is pregnant, has an STI, or has a history of PID. Because an IUD slightly increases the risk of PID, this type of EC is usually not recommended for women who want to bear children in the future. Side effects may include abdominal discomfort, vaginal bleeding or spotting, cramping, and infection.

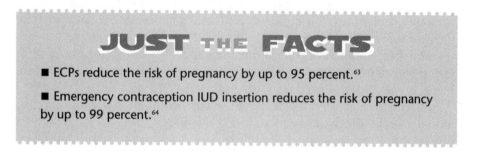

■ ECPs reduce the risk of pregnancy by up to 95 percent.[63]

■ Emergency contraception IUD insertion reduces the risk of pregnancy by up to 99 percent.[64]

EMERGENCY CONTRACEPTION HOTLINES

1-888-NOT-2-LATE
(1-888-668-2528)

Operated by the Princeton Office of Population Research in New Jersey and the Reproductive Health Technologies Project in Washington, D.C., this 24-hour hotline provides the names and numbers of clinicians in a caller's geographic area who prescribe EC. For more information, visit the Web site at *ec.princeton.edu.*

1-800-230-PLAN
(1-800-230-7526)

Call toll-free for a confidential appointment to arrange for EC at the nearest Planned Parenthood, or to schedule a pregnancy test. For more information, visit the Web site at *www.plannedparenthood.org.*

ABORTION

Approximately 1.4 million abortions are performed in the United States each year, which represents about one-third of all pregnancies (although abortions may be underreported).[65] Several abortion procedures are available, depending primarily on how advanced the pregnancy is, although different states allow different kinds of abortions. The earlier the abortion is performed, the simpler the procedure is, and the lower the risks are to the woman.

Some states have mandatory parental involvement laws, which require women under eighteen to tell a parent or get permission before having an abortion.

The most common way to terminate a pregnancy of up to twelve weeks (the first trimester) is vacuum aspiration, or the suction method. Fewer than 9 percent of abortions take place in the second trimester (weeks fourteen through twenty-four).[66] After twenty-four weeks, abortions are rare and done only for serious health reasons.

The drug mifepristone (formerly known as RU-486) has been used in Europe for many years as a pharmaceutical alternative to suction abortion. In 2000, the FDA approved it for use in the United States.

Mifepristone is used in combination with another drug (misoprostol) to end an early pregnancy, which the FDA defines as forty-nine days (seven weeks) since the woman's last menstrual period began.[67] Both are taken orally. In very low doses, mifepristone may also be used as emergency contraception (to prevent pregnancy) within five days of unprotected intercourse.[68] There are indications that mifepristone is safer than surgical abortion and may also be useful in the treatment of breast cancer, tumors of the brain and spinal cord, a disease of the adrenal glands, and endometriosis.[69]

Two drugs, methotrexate and misoprostol, can also be injected before the seventh week of fetal development. Some researchers believe this method requires less medical monitoring than mifepristone.[70]

Organizations like Planned Parenthood offer pregnancy counseling that explores the full range of options available to a pregnant woman. Faith-based counseling programs are also available.

Few aspects of sexuality are as controversial as abortion. Whatever your beliefs, share them with your teen and explain why you hold them. And listen to your teen as well. If ever your Adult needed to be in charge, this is the time. *

---

* See "The Miron Model" on pages 19–27.

What's Your Risk?

This questionnaire is for you. You don't have to show it to anyone else. It can help you determine whether you may be at risk for catching a sexually transmitted infection (STI). It can help you decide if you need more information or a medical checkup. IMPORTANT: *This questionnaire contains only basic information, and it is not the same as having a medical checkup.*

1. **Have you had sexual contact with another person—either mouth to genital, or genital to genital?** □ yes □ no

   If you answered **no**, you are not at risk. If you answered **yes**, go on to the next questions.

2. **Is he/she your first and only sexual partner?** □ yes □ no

3. **Are you his/her first and only sexual partner?** □ yes □ no □ don't know

   If you answered **yes** to both questions 2 and 3—and you're absolutely, positively sure about your partner—you are at low risk. Having sexual contact doesn't cause STIs. One person has to already have an infection to give it to someone else through sexual contact.

   If you answered **no** to question 2 and **yes** to question 3, you are not at risk—but your partner may be.

   If you answered **yes** to question 2 and **no** or **don't know** to question 3, you may be at risk. If you have sexual contact with someone who has had sexual contact with anyone else, there is some risk of catching an STI. Even one time may be enough. Many STIs cause no symptoms, particularly in women.

4. **Do you and your partner use protection during sexual contact—a latex condom and/or a dental dam?** □ never □ sometimes □ every time

   If you answered never or sometimes, you may be at risk.

Rate the Risk

Rate each of these behaviors according to the following scale:

A = Least Risky
B = Somewhat Risky
C = Risky
D = Dangerous

_____ Vaginal intercourse without a condom

_____ Talking, sharing fantasies

_____ Masturbation on skin that has no cuts, sores, or openings

_____ Open-mouthed kissing

_____ Masturbation on open sores or broken skin

_____ Oral sex with a latex barrier (condom or dental dam)

_____ Vaginal intercourse with a condom

_____ Oral sex without a latex barrier (condom or dental dam)

_____ Dry kissing

_____ Anal intercourse without a condom

_____ Massage or touching

_____ Anal intercourse with a condom

_____ Oral-anal contact without a latex barrier

Adapted from a questionnaire prepared by the McKinley Health Center, University of Illinois at Urbana-Champaign, © The Board of Trustees of the University of Illinois, 1995. Used with permission in *How to Talk with Teens About Love, Relationships, & S-E-X: A Guide for Parents* by Amy G. Miron, M.S., and Charles D. Miron, Ph.D., copyright © 2002, Free Spirit Publishing Inc., Minneapolis, MN; 866/703-7322; *www.freespirit.com*. This page may be photocopied for individual or small group use only.

Answers to "Rate the Risk" on page 202:

A—Least Risky
> Talking, sharing fantasies
> Dry kissing
> Massage or touching
> Masturbation on skin that has no cuts, sores or openings
> Oral sex with a latex barrier (condom or dental dam)

B—Somewhat Risky
> Open-mouthed kissing
> Vaginal intercourse with a condom
> Anal intercourse with a condom

C—Risky
> Oral sex without a latex barrier (condom or dental dam)
> Masturbation on open sores or broken skin

D—Dangerous
> Vaginal intercourse without a condom
> Anal intercourse without a condom
> Oral-anal contact without a latex barrier

Using a Condom

Choosing and Checking

1. Choose a latex condom with a receptacle tip. For oral sex, there are flavored condoms. For vaginal intercourse, there are condoms lubricated with nonoxynol-9. Don't confuse the two—anything that tastes good doesn't have the bitter but effective spermicide. Also, nonoxynol-9 can leave the tongue slightly numb.

2. Check the expiration date on the condom package. If the date has passed, throw the condom away and get a new one.

Putting It On

1. Open the package carefully—not with your teeth or a sharp object, which could tear the condom or put a hole in it. Watch for sharp fingernails, too. If you tear the condom, throw it away and get a new one. Don't open the package too far in advance. A condom can become dry and brittle within a few hours, causing it to tear easily.

2. Look at the condom to see which way it will unroll when placed over the erect penis. If placed on the penis inside-out, it won't roll down.

3. You may want to put a drop or two of water-based lubricant inside the condom or on the tip of the erect penis. Don't use too much lubricant or the condom may slide off.

4. Pinch the tip of the condom between the thumb and forefinger. (Think "pinch an inch.") This ensures that no air gets into the tip and there will be room at the end for the ejaculate. If you don't do this, the force of the ejaculation could rupture the latex and release the semen.

continued ⟶

Using a Condom continued

5. Before the penis comes into contact with any part of the other person's body, place the pinched end on the tip of the erect penis. Roll the condom down the shaft until it reaches the top of the scrotal sack, where the penis joins the man's body. Men who are uncircumcised should pull back the foreskin before unrolling the condom.

6. If the condom is not already lubricated on the outside by the manufacturer, lubricate it with a spermicide and/or a water-based lubricant. This reduces friction and helps prevent the condom from tearing. (Lubricant and spermicide can also be used on or in the other person.) Don't use an oil- or petroleum-based product (baby oil, cooking oil, hand lotion, or petroleum jelly). Oil weakens latex and can cause the condom to break.

Taking It Off

1. Immediately after ejaculation—*while the penis is still erect*—take hold of the rim of the condom at the base (the very bottom) of the penis. Firmly hold onto the rim and withdraw the penis from the other person's body. Holding onto the rim prevents the penis from sliding out of the condom during withdrawal. Sperm may drip out, so turn away from the other person's body.

2. Don't simply unroll the condom the way it was rolled on. Instead, grasp the rim of the condom with both hands at the base of the penis. Stretch the rim away from the penis. Lift it off the shaft, pulling it toward the tip of the penis. This protects the opening at the end of the penis from any secretions on the outside of the condom.

3. Tie the condom to contain the semen, or wrap it in a tissue or toilet paper before throwing it away. (Flushing a condom down the toilet could plug the pipes.) *A condom can only be used once.*

4. As a last step, both partners should wash their hands with soap and water. If possible, they should also urinate. While it's not foolproof, the acid in urine may help protect you from infections.

SEXUAL PLEASURE

Human beings have various emotions, needs, likes, dislikes, and responses. Not only are sexual arousal patterns different for different people, they're different for the same person at different times. What excites us on one day might not on the next.

You won't be able to flip through this chapter to find the magic formula for miraculous sex. It's not here. We're not holding out on you; it's just that technique is only part of the formula. It's useful to know a few basic facts about how human bodies work, but having enjoyable sex is much more about attitude and state of mind. No cookbook approach can help with that. But an open mind, mutual respect, good communication, and knowledge of himself and his partner can start your teen on the road to pleasurable sex for the rest of his life.

Like the rest of the information in this book, information about sexual pleasure is best when presented to your teen within the context of your value system. But all teens could benefit from knowing something about this topic, no matter what model of sexuality education you hold.

If you think that your teen should be abstinent until he's married, you could start your discussion about sexual pleasure with, "When you're married . . . ." If you want him to delay sexual expression until he's in a committed relationship, you could begin by saying, "When you and your fiancée . . . ." If you believe in responsible sexual expression, you could say, "When you and your partner . . . ."

You'll have to decide how much of this chapter to share with your teen. Before you conclude that a particular fact or issue is inappropriate, remember that negative messages about sex can be hard to unlearn later in life. In our practice, we've seen many people who received strong negative messages about sexuality throughout their younger years. As married adults, they had trouble making good sexual connections with their partners.

Keep in mind that the absence of a message may be heard as a negative message. What are you telling your teen if you teach him about sexually transmitted infections (STIs) and pregnancy prevention, but you never even mention sexual pleasure?

In "Step 1: Define Your Goals and Values," a "Try This" exercise asked you to list the goals you have for your teen as a fully sexually educated young adult.* Look back at those goals now. Most of us want our teens to enjoy the varied pleasures that responsible sexual expression can bring—when the time is right. To help your teen reach that goal, talk with him about the joys and pleasures of sex, as well as its risks and consequences. You can emphasize that the more emotionally mature and prepared he is, the more he will enjoy sex.

You might also tell your teen that the brain is nature's best aphrodisiac. What makes sex enjoyable—or not—most often takes place between our ears. When we have any reservations about our sexual behavior, our mind is likely to block our sexual enjoyment or arousal level. If a man feels pressured to engage in sexual activity that he isn't emotionally ready for, he may lose his erection. If a woman isn't emotionally ready for sex, her mental tensions can translate to body tension, which can block orgasm or make sexual intercourse painful.

Love with the Perfect Stranger?

Teens are constantly bombarded with unrealistic messages about love and sex. Books, songs, TV, and movies present them with images of sexual relationships that begin when two strangers glance across the room.

Their eyes lock. Slowly, they drift toward each other, mesmerized. Before long, they leave together. Outside the door, they begin kissing. They fall across the back seat of the car, tearing at each other's clothes. Within minutes, they both experience wild, exquisite orgasms (with no protection, of course). After that, they might pause long enough to learn each other's names.

With a few minor changes here and there, that's the scenario for the beginning of a wonderful love affair—in the movies. In real life, it's ridiculous as well as risky. Teens who buy into this sex-sex fantasy** are going to be sorely disappointed. In fact, this is a pretty fair summary of how *not* to have a good sexual experience.

If you and your teen are watching a TV show or movie when a version of the above scenario takes place, you have a perfect opportunity to begin a conversation. (Don't interrupt a show your teen is engrossed in, though. Wait for a commercial or the show's end.) Let your teen know that one of the many things wrong with the stranger fantasy is that a gorgeous stranger is still a stranger. Explain that while looks may lure her in, personality, friendship, and common interests count for more.

---

* Find this exercise on page 13.

** See "Love-Sex, Fun-Sex, and Sex-Sex" on pages 16–17.

You might also mention that an intimate and sexual relationship can grow out of a friendship. Your teen may find that she's become crazy about someone she never expected to be physically attracted to—all because she likes that person so much in other ways.

Let your teen know that she's unlikely to experience great sex with a person she doesn't know well. Remind her of how awkward conversation can be with someone she barely knows. If talking is awkward, imagine how much more uncomfortable a sexual experience would be. Teach your teen that the great love-sex you hope she'll have sometime in her life is a shared experience. It takes mutual respect, communication, commitment, knowledge of herself and her partner, time, affection, and openness to each other as people—not just as sex objects.

It is possible to have great sex-sex with a stranger. But it's also possible to get hit by lightning—and it's often just as dangerous.

Sexual Fantasies

Most people have sexual fantasies, including your teen. How you feel about them will depend on your values, but teens need to know that just because they have a fantasy about something doesn't mean they'd necessarily want to try it. Thought and action are two different things.

If you believe that sexual thoughts or fantasies are wrong, talk with your teen. Let him know what you think and why. If you believe that sexual fantasy is acceptable, find a teachable moment to address the topic. For example, when you see someone daydreaming on TV or in real life, you could say something like, "Don't you wonder what that person is daydreaming about? I wonder if he's having a sexual fantasy." If that gets a snicker or a laugh, you could say, "What's so funny? Most people have sexual fantasies," and then discuss your views on the topic.

JUST THE FACTS

- Researchers found that 54 percent of men and 19 percent of women said that they thought about sex at least once a day.[1]

- A study of 212 married college women found that 88 percent had sexual fantasies both during masturbation and sexual intercourse.[2]

You might explain that erotic imaginings can make for great entertainment during fun-sex or sex-sex, values permitting. If your teen believes in an abstinence or delay model, sharing fantasies with a partner can be an alternative to intercourse. At the right time, with the right person, acting out a fantasy together can also be exciting. However, both partners need to be in agreement about the fantasy. If either partner is uncomfortable, it won't be a positive experience.

Tell your teen that some people aren't interested in sharing or acting out sexual fantasies. That's another one of those individual preferences that needs to be respected.

Sexual Arousal and Response

A surprising number of teens, even those who have had sex education classes in school, are ignorant about the physical and sexual responses of the other sex—or their own sex. Often, sexual arousal and response aren't even covered in sex education.

JUST THE FACTS

■ In one series of national surveys, students said that their most recent sex education course included information about "core elements" (HIV/AIDS, abstinence, STDs, and the basics of reproduction) and "other topics" (birth control, abortion, sexual orientation and homosexuality). Sexual arousal and response weren't listed in either category.[3]

■ The Sexuality Information and Education Council of the United States (SIECUS) recommends that human sexual response be part of a comprehensive sexuality education program, starting with simple messages in middle childhood ("Both boys and girls may discover that their bodies feel good when touched") and adding more specific details in early adolescence and adolescence.[4]

Scientific understanding of what actually goes on in men's and women's bodies during sexual activity is relatively new.[5] William Masters and Virginia Johnson, followed by many other researchers, have found that, physically, men and women both go through a series of four phases: arousal, plateau, orgasm, and resolution. The timing of these phases is different for men and women, but both sexes journey through the same basic sequence.

In the best scenario, the journey begins with mutual desire on the part of both partners. Desire leads to activities that build arousal. During this phase, sexual excitement causes vaginal lubrication in the woman and erection in the man. As sexual stimulation continues, a woman's clitoris enlarges, her labia open and increase in size, her vagina lengthens and widens, and her breasts swell. A man's testicles increase in size and become elevated. Muscle tension, blood pressure, respiratory rate, and heart rate increase for both sexes.

With continued sexual activity, both women and men enter the plateau phase. A woman's clitoris begins to pull back under the clitoral hood. A man's penis becomes fully erect, and his Cowper's glands secrete pre-ejaculatory fluid. The skin of both women and men sometimes takes on a rosy flush, and their nipples may become erect. There is a further increase of muscle tension, blood pressure, respiratory rate, and heart rate.

With more stimulation, both women and men can experience an orgasm, the sudden pleasurable release of built-up sexual tension. Women will have vaginal and uterine contractions. Men will ejaculate. After orgasm (or eventually, if orgasm has not occurred), the bodies of both women and men will return to their pre-arousal state—the resolution phase. The uterus and clitoris return to their normal positions. The penis returns to its normal flaccid state.

Men will go through a refractory period, during which they can't respond to sexual stimulation. This period may be so short as to go unnoticed in teens, but it will gradually lengthen as men grow older. Regardless of their age, women don't have a refractory period. If they want, they can go right into the next sexual cycle without waiting.

This is the scientific understanding of human sexual arousal and response, in brief. On paper, it sounds straightforward. In person, it can be complicated, confusing, and even frightening—especially for someone who's engaging in sexual activity for the first time.

For example, most men are very familiar with their own penises. After all, they handle them several times a day when urinating, showering, or masturbating. They don't understand why touching or stroking one should be such a big deal to a woman. To an inexperienced woman, however, the penis—especially in its erect state—is an alien object. She may wonder if, when, and how to touch it.

Tell your teen that good sex requires good communication. She needs to be able to ask her partner what pleases him, and to explain what pleases her. Demonstrating is another way of letting her partner know what she'd like done and how, although it's not wise to rely solely on nonverbal communication.

A young woman may also wonder what to do with testicles. She's probably heard that hitting or squeezing them causes great pain. Should she touch them at all? If so, how? The answer is as unique as the person who owns them. If your daughter asks, "What about a guy's testicles? If you're fooling around, should you play with them?" you might answer, "Some men like to have them played with, but others don't. It's another one of those personal things. You need to be able to talk with your partner to find out how he feels about it."

To an inexperienced man, the vagina can seem even more alien than a penis does to a woman. A man's genitals are easy to read. When a man is sexually aroused, his penis stands up. When he's not, it doesn't. In contrast, a woman's vagina is mysterious and hidden. A man can't engage in sexual inter-course unless he is aroused—but a woman can. A vagina can be receptive to intercourse even if not aroused, although intercourse will probably be painful.

Both young men and young women are likely to know little to nothing about the clitoris, because it's seldom talked about. The clitoris is extremely sensitive and exists for no other known reason than to give a woman sexual pleasure. By withholding this information from our teens, we may be fos-tering the double standard, implying that sexual pleasure is okay for men but not for women.

Consider how odd it would be for a man to engage in sexual contact with little or no stimulation of his penis. For many women, the clitoris—the female equivalent of the penis—is largely ignored, even though stimulation of the clitoris is the most common source of their arousal and orgasm.

The clitoris changes as a woman's sexual arousal increases. Initially, the clitoris is up front and prominent. With continued arousal, it retracts under the clitoral hood. This means that the pattern of stimulation that was pleas-ing in the early phase of sexual response may not be pleasing later on. The woman's partner needs to ask about this, listen to the answers, and tune into nonverbal cues.

The inside of the vagina is relatively insensitive. Most of a woman's sex-ual arousal comes from stimulation of the clitoris and labia, as well as other parts of her body that she finds arousing. What other parts? This varies from woman to woman. Some women can be aroused and even brought to orgasm by stimulation of a spot on the upper front wall of the vagina. In other women, this area is less sensitive. It's called the G-spot, after German obstetrician and gynecologist Ernest Gräfenberg, who first wrote about it.

People who are aroused by women's breasts may be puzzled when something they find so exciting provides little or no arousal for their partner. Some women are excited by having their breasts attended to; others aren't. And to make it even more confusing for her partner, a woman's breasts may be tender during some stages of her menstrual cycle. Because of her chang-ing hormones, what feels good one day may hurt some days later. Again, communication is key.

Kissing is another source of sexual arousal. Teens often ask, "What's the right way to kiss?" Here again, each person is different. Some people enjoy wet kisses. Others hate them. Some like one continuous, long kiss. Others prefer short, intermittent kisses. Some people find firm kisses arousing. Others like tender kisses. And, of course, there's the question of what to do with your tongue, which is another of those personal preference issues. Also, the kind of kissing a person was in the mood for yesterday may be quite dif-ferent from what he'd like today.

Watching a movie or TV will usually present an opportunity to initiate a discussion about kissing with your teen. You could point out how different actors are kissing in different ways in different scenes. If your teen asks, "What's the right way to kiss?" you could say, "Your lips should be saying what your heart is feeling." Or, "Bad kissers are people who don't let their feelings come through their lips." Or, "What you're in the mood for sexually can change."

Gay, lesbian, bisexual, and transgendered (GLBT) teens also wonder how to stimulate each other's bodies. Just because you own a similar set of genitals doesn't mean you know how to pleasure them. Most media images of love and sex show heterosexual couples. GLBT teens don't have as much access to models of arousal. If you and your GLBT teen are watching TV or a movie showing a heterosexual flirtation or love scene, you might say, "Isn't it sad that they don't show gay or lesbian couples being romantic?" Or, "Pleasing your partner is about communicating. It doesn't matter whether you're gay or straight."

Your teen may have heard that once a man reaches a certain point of arousal, he has to have an orgasm or he'll suffer excruciating pain. There's even a slang name for this: "blue balls." It's a myth. If a man is sexually aroused for a prolonged period of time, it's true that his testicles can become painful, although they don't turn blue. But orgasm is not the only way to get relief. Once the erection subsides, the tenderness will go away.

This phenomenon isn't exclusive to males. A similar thing happens to a women's vulva after extended sexual arousal without sexual release. The fact that we don't have a slang name for this shows how little attention our society pays to female sexuality.

We've focused here on understanding a partner's sexual responses, but teens also need to understand their own responses. Human sexual arousal has four sources: touching your partner's body for your pleasure; having your partner touch your body; experiencing your partner's growing arousal; and sexual fantasy. The more sources of arousal that are used, the more exciting the sexual experience will be.

Traditionally, men have been more comfortable than women about using all four sources of arousal. Many women attend to their partner's body primarily to provide pleasure for their partner, not themselves. (That's called work, not pleasure.) Women need to learn how to use their partner's body for their own pleasure, and that it's okay to do so.

Orgasm

Teens often wonder what an orgasm feels like. When we're asked, we offer an analogy: It feels like a sneeze. We suggest that the teen think about a time when she had a tickle in her nose and felt she had to sneeze. The tension of the tickle built up and up—until she finally sneezed. What a relief!

An orgasm has that same build-up of tension, only it's sexual tension. It's followed by a sudden release, which feels very good.

An orgasm is a total body experience. Respiration, heart rate, and blood pressure reach their peak. Toes may point, heads may toss back, breath is often held. A women's uterus will contract rhythmically, along with the inside of her vagina. A man's prostate, seminal vesicles, and urethral bulb contract, expelling semen.

Both women and men experience a sudden release of sexual tension, accompanied by a pleasurable feeling. While all orgasms feel good, they are not all created equal. Some are very intense. Others are nothing to write home about.

Some young women fear having an orgasm because they associate it with losing control. When they hear about all of the physiological things that happen during orgasm, the idea of having one themselves may scare them. If you sense that your daughter is afraid of what's going to happen when (or if) she has an orgasm, you could explain that orgasms feel good— they're a positive thing. True, a few muscles contract, and she can't control them (just like when her eye twitches), but this doesn't mean that *she* is out of control.

In a stereotypical fantasy of sexual intercourse between a man and a woman, both partners experience wild and rapid arousal. Receiving the penis into the vagina sends the woman into shrieks of ecstasy. It all culminates quickly in earth-shaking simultaneous orgasms.

That's the fantasy, not the reality—but it's such a common belief that many women fake orgasm during intercourse just to please their partners. They're embarrassed that they're taking so long. They think there's something wrong with them, or they worry that their partner will think there's something wrong. In fact, men and women have a different timeline to their sexual responses. Most women take a lot longer than most men to reach orgasm, and they require a lot more stimulation. That's just the way women are built. The more sources of arousal a woman has access to, the more she's likely to shorten the time she needs to reach orgasm.

Simultaneous orgasms can be fun, but they take patience, practice, experimentation, coordination, and knowledge of yourself, your partner, and the sexual responses of both people. With time, a couple can learn to judge each other's responses reasonably well, but this rarely happens outside of committed long-term relationships.

In heterosexual intercourse, the friction generated by the penis rubbing against the walls of the vagina is what commonly causes an orgasm for the male. Many men—and women—assume that this friction will provide enough stimulation for the female to reach an orgasm as well. But for many women, that's not how it works. Most heterosexual women find pleasure in vaginal intercourse, but it's often not the source of orgasm. What will most likely bring a woman to orgasm is direct stimulation of her clitoris, along with the other parts of her body that she finds pleasurable.

Most women enjoy prolonged foreplay, including kissing and touching of the body—the whole body, not just the clitoris and vagina. Foreplay often includes the talking and sharing that precedes and occurs during the sexual experience. Most men also enjoy foreplay and talking before sexual intercourse. Many people, male as well as female, need to feel connected and attended to, if not loved, by their partner in order to have a positive sexual experience.

Many sexual activities can bring men and women to orgasm. For women, attending to the parts of her body that she finds pleasurable, and stimulating the clitoris long enough with a hand, mouth, penis, or vibrator, will probably bring her to orgasm. Exactly how to best stimulate a clitoris (or any part of her body) will vary from woman to woman. Some like a firm touch; others don't. Some enjoy a circular pattern of stimulation; others prefer an up-and-down motion. Some women like lots of pressure; others don't. Some women like having their ears nibbled; others can't stand that activity. Again, it's a personal thing, and it can change with the same woman on different occasions.

For most men, stimulating any part of his body that he finds pleasurable while attending to his penis with a hand, mouth, or vagina will probably lead to an orgasm. How and where to stimulate the penis and the rest of the man's body is a personal thing. Some men like short, fast movements over the shaft and glans; others like a long, slow, teasing touch. For both sexes, what works best is asking and experimenting together. This is all part of an intimate relationship.

Teens often have questions about the timing of orgasms. If your teen approaches you with questions, be glad that you have the kind of relationship where he feels comfortable talking with you about personal issues. Then answer him as openly and honestly as you can.

WHAT TO SAY?

If your teen asks . . .
"What if I have an orgasm too soon?" or "What if I take too long?"

You might say . . .
"Good sex isn't on a schedule. You need to know yourself and your partner and communicate with each other about what's pleasing. Each partner and each experience is different and will take different amounts of time."

continued ⟶

If your teen asks . . .
"What's a 'minute man'? Why is that so funny?"

You might say . . .
"A 'minute man' is a guy who ejaculates after a minute's worth of sexual stimulation. Many men reach orgasm quickly. It's pretty common. With time and experience, a man can learn to slow down his response. Some people laugh and make jokes about common things that they're uncomfortable with."

If your teen asks . . .
"Why is it so hard for a girl to have an orgasm?"

You might say . . .
"Women are wired differently than men. Most women require more time and more stimulation than men do to experience an orgasm."

You might add . . .
"The more a woman worries about the amount of time she's taking, the less likely she is to concentrate on her sources of arousal. When that happens, she may not be able to have an orgasm at all."

Or you might say . . .
"With time, knowledge about each other, and experience, it sometimes gets quicker."

Erotica

Erotica isn't the same as pornography. Erotica is sexually arousing material—books, magazines, movies, videos, audio recordings, Web sites, and so on—that is not considered obscene or offensive to the average person. It also has goals other than sexual arousal; it may be part of artistic expression. Pornography is sexually arousing material that is considered obscene and offensive, and its only goal is sexual arousal.

Of course, what's obscene and offensive to one person might not be to another—and vice versa. And who is the "average person," anyway? Battles have raged for centuries around these issues, and they'll probably keep raging for centuries more.

What if you find an X-rated magazine in your teen's room? ("Find" as in "discover by accident" in the course of a normal activity, such as changing bed linens—not "find" as in "discover while snooping.") First, stay calm. Almost all teens eventually look at X-rated magazines. You probably looked at them yourself. Second, decide what you want to do. Put the magazine back where you found it and say nothing? Or tell your teen about your discovery, then talk about it openly? Maybe that depends on the magazine. Hard-core pornography is one thing; something like *Playboy* may be another.

If you choose to talk with your teen, you might say, "I found [name of magazine] in your room today." If you don't approve, you can follow by saying, "I don't want X-rated magazines in our home. Please get rid of it." Or you might say, "I understand that you're curious about men's and women's bodies and sex. Curiosity is normal. Lots of people look at magazines like the one I found in your room. I hope you'll come to me with any questions you have."

What if the magazine you found belongs to you or your partner? Deal with the privacy issue first. Was your teen snooping through your things? That's not acceptable. Or was the magazine left out in the open for anyone to find? If you don't want your teen reading X-rated magazines, perhaps you shouldn't have them in the house—or if you do, you should keep them where your teen isn't likely to find them, by accident or on purpose.

If you talk with your teen about erotica, you might start by explaining the difference between erotica and pornography. Then, depending on your values, you could say something like this: "A lot of people find erotica sexually arousing. Reading books or magazines, looking at pictures, watching videos, or sharing erotic fantasies can be exciting. For many couples, erotica is part of their sex play. But some people don't find it interesting at all. And some people find it offensive. It's a personal thing, and people are different."

Sex Toys

Many products supposedly enhance the sexual experience, and your teen may have heard about some of them. We're providing the following information so that if you're questioned, you'll have answers if you want to give them. We think it's better for your curious teen to get this information from you rather than from a magazine advertisement promoting a ridiculous product, or from an uninformed (or misinformed) friend.

The most common sex toy is probably the vibrator. Vibrators are just what their name says—objects that vibrate. They can be battery operated or electric and come in a variety of shapes and sizes. Some can be used for tired muscles anywhere on the body. Some include removable attachments that are designed for stimulating specific parts of the body—like the head, neck, lower back, or genitals. A vibrator shaped like a penis is made to be used on the clitoris or in the vagina. Many women report that the use of a vibrator intensifies their orgasms. While men can use them on the underside of the penis, we've found few who do.

Dildos—penis-shaped cylinders—have existed for centuries. They can be made of almost anything, but modern dildos are commonly made of flexible plastic. They are used most often during masturbation, but can be used with a partner as well. A dildo that's going to be inserted into a body should be lubricated with a water-based lubricant. This is critical if the dildo will be used in the anus, since there's no natural lubrication in that area of the body. Also, a dildo used in the anal area should have a flanged base so it doesn't slip inside. Once a dildo (or anything, for that matter) has been inserted into the anal area, it must be washed well with soap and water before being used vaginally.

Condoms can be used to cover vibrators, dildos, and other sex toys that are inserted into the body. A fresh condom should be used for each partner and each part of the body. Flavored condoms and dental dams have been created to add fun to the experience of oral sex. They also protect against STIs.

Hot oils, body paints, and sexy lingerie can add spice to sexual relationships. Oils and lotions should not be used inside the body. Only water-based lubricants are intended for internal use. They can also be used externally, to increase sexual pleasure and fun.

Some of the sex-aid products on the market are nothing more than sexual snake oil. The claims made by their manufacturers are either greatly exaggerated or downright false, and some of the products are dangerous. For example, creams to slow down a man's orgasm seldom work and can be harmful. They may contain chemicals that cause a rash, burning, irritation, and infection of the urethra.

Cock rings, which are usually made of metal or plastic, encircle the base of the penis to keep it erect longer. They prevent the blood that has flowed into the penis during arousal from flowing back into the body. Because they impair circulation, they can cause problems if worn too tightly or left on for too long. A cock ring should not be so loose that it slips off before erection—or so tight that the wearer can't get it off during erection.

Ben-Wa balls, which are usually made of metal, are placed in the vagina. When a woman rocks back and forth, they're supposed to keep her sexually aroused. Like any object inserted into the vagina, they should be cleaned before and after use. They should not be left in the body for a prolonged period of time.

Some sexual partners use a cord that has a knot or bead every inch or so and a ring at one end. After a water-based lubricant is applied, the cord is inserted into the anus with the ring hanging out. At the moment of orgasm, the ring is pulled and the string is withdrawn. The knots or beads are supposed to enhance orgasm. This toy must be washed well with soap and water between uses (as must both partners' hands) so that fecal material is not passed on.

If you talk with your teens about sex toys, encourage them to use common sense. You might want to say that nature has already provided us with all the equipment we'll ever need for a lifetime of great sex. Not only do we possess wonderful sex organs, we have inventive minds, creative imaginations, strong emotions, and a sense of humor. With both partners accessing all those assets, the sky's the limit.

A FEW FINAL WORDS

Talking with teens about love, relationships, and sex isn't such a tough task once you're prepared. We hope we've provided some information, insights, and strategies that will help you and your teen discuss these difficult issues—if not entirely comfortably, then at least openly and honestly, within the context of your values and beliefs.

Just as Rome wasn't built in a day, neither should the sexuality education of your teen be a sudden or hurried process. Many little talks inspired by teachable moments are much more productive than one "big talk."

Take care to nurture your relationship with your teen. Let your Child come out and play with your teen's Child. Let your Adolescent come out and play with your teen's Adolescent. Just make sure that your Adult is in charge when you and your teen are talking about love, relationships, and sex.

You are the most important educator your child will ever have. Even if you don't think you're an "expert" on sex, you can teach your teen what he or she needs to know to make healthy, positive, responsible choices. If you've read this book, you have a good working knowledge of topics you might cover and words you might use.

Don't worry about not getting everything right. Don't be surprised if you still feel uneasy or embarrassed at times, or if you fall back into old patterns and habits you're trying to change. That's how people grow—two steps forward, one step back. You might even want to point this out to your teen. Please don't let your discomfort stop you from continuing his or her sexuality education.

And don't be discouraged if your teen doesn't immediately respond the way you'd like. It takes time and consistency for new patterns to change the old dynamics in any relationship. Keep your Adult in charge, and try to communicate about what you feel. It's a learning process for both you and your teen. Give yourselves time.

You may want to keep this book around and refer back to it as issues arise. Rereading something can often bring new and deeper understandings of the material.

We're open to your comments, opinions, and suggestions. We'd love to hear your stories. You may contact us in care of our publisher:

Free Spirit Publishing Inc.
217 Fifth Avenue North, Suite 200
Minneapolis, MN 55401-1299
help4kids@freespirit.com

We wish you and your family the best in your journeys.

NOTES

Introduction

1. J. Dryfoos, "What the United States Can Learn About Prevention of Teenage Pregnancy from Other Developed Countries," *SIECUS Reports* 14, 1–7 (November 1985).

2. L.S. Zabin, et al., "Adolescent Pregnancy Prevention Program: A Model for Research and Evaluation," *Journal of Adolescent Health Care* 7, 77–87 (1986); L.S. Zabin, et al., "Evaluation of a Pregnancy Prevention Program for Urban Teenagers," *Family Planning Perspectives* 18:3, 119–126 (1986); L.S. Zabin, et al., "The Baltimore Pregnancy Prevention Program for Urban Adolescents: How Did It Work?" *Family Planning Perspectives* 20:4, 182–187 (1988).

3. B.C. Miller, *Families Matter: A Research Synthesis of Family Influences on Adolescent Pregnancy* (Washington, DC: National Campaign to Prevent Teen Pregnancy, 1998).

4. M.K. Hutchinson and T.M. Cooney, "Patterns of Parent-Teen Sexual Risk Communication: Implications for Intervention," *Family Relations* 47, 185–194 (1998).

5. "Teenage Pregnancy: Overall Trends and State-by-State Information" (New York: The Alan Guttmacher Institute, 1999).

6. "Fact Sheet: Recent Trends in Teen Pregnancy and Birth, Sexual Activity, and Contraceptive Use" (Washington, DC: National Campaign to Prevent Teen Pregnancy, August 2001).

7. American Social Health Association, "Sexually Transmitted Diseases in America: How Many Cases and at What Cost?" (Menlo Park, CA: Kaiser Family Foundation, December 1998).

8. *Sex and America's Teenagers* (New York: The Alan Guttmacher Institute, 1994).

9. *Sex and America's Teenagers* (New York: The Alan Guttmacher Institute, 1994).

10. "Youth Risk Behavior Surveillance—United States, 1999," *CDC/MMWR Surveillance Summaries* 49:SS05 1–96 (June 9, 2000).

11. L.S. Stepp, "Parents Are Alarmed by an Unsettling New Fad in Middle Schools: Oral Sex," *Washington Post* (July 8, 1999).

12. J. Wasserhut, M.D., American Association of Sex Educators, Counselors and Therapists (AASECT) National Convention Workshop (1997).

13. "Risky Business: A 2000 Poll: Teens Tell Us What They Really Think of Contraception and Sex" (Washington, DC: National Campaign to Prevent Teen Pregnancy, 2000).

14. E.O. Laumann, et al., *The Social Organization of Sexuality: Sexual Practices in the United States* (Chicago: University of Chicago Press, 1994).

Step 1: Define Your Values and Goals

1. "Decision Making," a publication of the SexSmarts public information partnership between the Kaiser Family Foundation and *seventeen* magazine (September 2000).

2. "Talking with Teens: The YMCA Parent and Teen Survey Final Report" (Chicago: YMCA of the USA, 2000).

Step 2: Understand Your Teen's Personality

1. D. Kunkel, et al., "Sex on TV (2): A Biennial Report to the Kaiser Family Foundation" (Menlo Park, CA: Kaiser Family Foundation, 2001).

2. C.L. Perry, et al., "The Social World of Adolescents: Family Peers, Schools and the Community." In *Promoting the Health of Adolescents: New Directions for the Twenty-first Century*, edited by S. Millstein, et al., 73–97 (New York: Oxford University Press, 1993).

Step 3: Understand Your Teen's Sexual Development

1. J. Willis, "On the Teen Scene: Acne Agony" (Washington, DC: U.S. Food and Drug Administration, 1999).

2. R.W. Blum and P.M. Rinehart, *Reducing the Risk: Connections That Make a Difference in the Lives of Youth* (Minneapolis: University of Minnesota, Department of Pediatrics, 1997).

Step 4: Understand Your Teen's Relationships

1. P. Bearman, et al., *Peer Potential: Making the Most of How Teens Influence Each Other* (Washington, DC: The National Campaign to Prevent Teen Pregnancy, 1999).

2. "Decision Making," a publication of the SexSmarts public information partnership between the Kaiser Family Foundation and *seventeen* magazine (September 2000).

3. P. Bearman and H. Bruckner, *Power in Numbers: Peer Effects on Adolescent Girls' Sexual Debut and Pregnancy* (Washington, DC: The National Campaign to Prevent Teen Pregnancy, 1999).

4. J.G. Silverman, et al., "Dating Violence Against Adolescent Girls and Associated Substance Use, Unhealthy Weight Control, Sexual Risk Behavior, Pregnancy and Suicidality," *Journal of the American Medical Association* 286:5, 572–579 (2001).

5. M. Jonson-Reid and L. Bivens, "Foster youth and dating violence," *Journal of Interpersonal Violence* 14:2, 1249–1262 (1999).

6. "Youth Risk Behavior Surveillance—United States, 1999," *CDC/MMWR Surveillance Summaries* 49:SS05, 1–96 (June 9, 2000).

7. V.A. Foshee, et al., "The Safe Dates Project: Theoretical Basis, Evaluation Design, and Selected Baseline Findings," *The Prevention Researcher* 7, 5–7 (2000); K. Powell and D. Hawkins, eds., "Youth Violence Prevention: Description and Baseline Data from 13 Evaluation Projects," *American Journal of Preventive Medicine*, Supplements 12:5, 39–47 (1996).

8. "Social Control, Verbal Abuse, and Violence Among Teenagers" (Washington, DC: The Empower Program/Liz Claiborne Inc., February 2001).

9. K.A. Moore and A. Driscoll, *Not Just for Girls: The Role of Boys and Men in Teen Pregnancy Prevention* (Washington, DC: The National Campaign to Prevent Teen Pregnancy and Child Trends, Inc., 1997).

10. D.A. Glei, "Measuring Contraceptive Use Patterns Among Teenage and Adult Women," *Family Planning Perspectives* 32:6, 295–297, 304 (1999).

11. "Decision Making," a publication of the SexSmarts public information partnership between the Kaiser Family Foundation and *seventeen* magazine (September 2000).

12. American Psychiatric Association, *Diagnostic and Statistical Manual of Mental Disorders*, 4th ed. (Washington, DC: American Psychiatric Association, 1994).

13. The danger signs of suicide were compiled by Tracy Pierson. Copyright © 1995–2000 SAVE (Suicide Awareness Voices of Education). SAVE gives permission to copy and use, in its entirety, any and all of the information on its Web site with SAVE and author credits. On the Web: www.save.org.

Step 5: Choose Your Model and Customize It

1. N. Shook, et al., "Courtship Violence Among College Students: A Comparison of Verbally and Physically Abusive Couples," *Journal of Family Violence* 15, 1–22 (2000).

2. U.S. Department of Health and Human Services, "National Survey Results on Drug Use from the Monitoring the Future Study, 1975–1995: Vol.1., Secondary School Students," (Washington, DC: U.S. Government Printing Office, 1997).

3. B. Flanigan, et al., "Alcohol Use as a Situational Influence on Young Women's Pregnancy Risk-Taking Behaviors," *Adolescence* 25, 205–214 (1990).

4. D.B. Kandel, "Early Onset of Adolescent Sexual Behavior and Drug Involvement," *Journal of Marriage and the Family* 52, 783–798 (1990).

5. Ibid.

6. "Decision Making," a publication of the SexSmarts public information partnership between the Kaiser Family Foundation and *seventeen* magazine (September 2000).

7. Peter S. Bearman and Hannah Brückner, "Promising the Future: Virginity Pledges and First Intercourse," *American Journal of Sociology* 106:4, 859–912 (January 2001).

8. *Sex Education in America: A View from Inside the Nation's Classrooms* (Menlo Park, CA: Kaiser Family Foundation, September 2000).

Step 6: Talk with Your Teen

1. "Talking with Teens: The YMCA Parent and Teen Survey Final Report" (Chicago: YMCA of the USA, 2000).

2. Ibid.

3. D. Schnarch, *Passionate Marriage* (New York: Norton, 1997).

Step 7: Be Prepared for Almost Anything

1. "Fact Sheet: Recent Trends in Teen Pregnancy and Birth, Sexual Activity, and Contraceptive Use" (Washington, DC: National Campaign to Prevent Teen Pregnancy, August 2001).

2. Ibid.

3. Ibid.

4. *Hostile Hallways: Bullying, Teasing, and Sexual Harassment in School* (Washington, DC: American Association of University Women Educational Foundation, 2001).

5. Ibid.

6. Ibid.

7. *Making Schools Safe for Gay and Lesbian Youth* (Boston: The Governor's Commission on Gay and Lesbian Youth, 1993).

8. Ibid.

9. Dr. Karen Franklin to the American Psychological Association, August 1998; cited in "From Our House to the Schoolhouse: Families & Educators Partnering for Safe Schools" (Washington, DC: PFLAG, 2000).

10. P. Cameron, et al., "Child Molestation and Homosexuality," *Psychological Reports* 58, 327–337 (1986).

11. D. Finkelhor, et al., "Sexual Abuse in a National Survey of Adult Men and Women: Prevalence, Characteristics and Risk Factors," *Child Abuse and Neglect* 14, 19–28 (1990).

12. "Youth Risk Behavior Surveillance—United States, 1999," *CDC/MMWR Surveillance Summaries* 49:SS05, 1–96 (June 9, 2000).

13. C. Ringel, "Criminal Victimization 1996: Changes 1995–96 with Trends 1993–96," National Crime Victimization Survey, 1996, NCJ-165812 (Washington, DC: Bureau of Justice Statistics, U.S. Department of Justice, November 1997); "Criminal Victimization in the United States, 1996 Statistical Tables" (Washington, DC: Bureau of Justice Statistics, U.S. Department of Justice, 1997).

14. "Criminal Victimization in the United States, 1997 Statistical Tables" (Washington, DC: Bureau of Justice Statistics, U.S. Department of Justice, 1998).

15. C. Bohmer and A. Parrot, *Sexual Assault on Campus: The Problem and the Solution* (New York: Lexington Books, 1993).

16. P. Tjaden and N. Thoennes, Stalking in America: Findings from the National Violence Against Women Survey (Washington, DC: National Institute of Justice, U.S. Department of Justice, April 1998).

17. Stalking (Washington, DC: National Center for Victims of Crime, 1995).

Issue 1: Female Sexual Development

1. C. Etaugh and S.A. Rathus, *The World of Children* (Fort Worth, TX: Harcourt Brace College Publishers, 1995).

2. Information from: R.M. Malina and C. Bouchard, *Growth, Maturation, and Physical Activity* (Champaign, IL: Human Kinetics, 1991); J.M. Tanner, *Foetus into Man* (Cambridge, MA: Harvard University Press, 1990); and L.E. Berk, *Infants, Children, and Adolescents* (Needham Heights, MA: Allyn & Bacon, 1999).

3. Facts About Eating Disorders (Highland Park, IL: National Association of Anorexia Nervosa and Associated Disorders, 2000).

4. Ibid.

5. 2000 National Plastic Surgery Statistics: Cosmetic and Reconstructive Plastic Surgery (Arlington Heights, IL: American Society of Plastic Surgeons, 2001).

6. H. Zoller, Leading the Fight Against Breast Cancer, *Cancer News* 47:1, 4—5 (1993).

7. N. Baxter with the Canadian Task Force on Preventive Health Care, Preventive Health Care, 2001 Update: Should Women Be Routinely Taught Breast Self-examination to Screen for Breast Cancer? *Canadian Medical Association Journal* 164:13, 1837—46 (2001).

Issue 2: Male Sexual Development

1. Steroids: Play Safe, Play Fair (Elk Grove Village, IL: American Academy of Pediatrics, 2001).

2. Ibid.

3. Information from: R.M. Malina and C. Bouchard, *Growth, Maturation, and Physical Activity* (Champaign, IL: Human Kinetics, 1991); J.M. Tanner, *Foetus into Man* (Cambridge, MA: Harvard University Press, 1990); and L.E. Berk, *Infants, Children, and Adolescents* (Needham Heights, MA: Allyn & Bacon, 1999).

4. B. Wolf, Penis Survey Comes Up Short (ABC News Internet Ventures, 2001).

5. Penis Size Survey conducted and reported at the Durex Scientific Web site: *www.durex.com.*

6. Penis Size Survey conducted by and reported at *www.altpenis.com.*

7. J.L. Stanford, et al., Prostate Cancer Trends 1973—1995, SEER Program, National Cancer Institute, NIH Pub. No. 99-4543 (Bethesda, MD: National Cancer Institute, 1999).

Issue 3: Sexual Orientation

1. E.O. Laumann, et al., *The Social Organization of Sexuality: Sexual Practices in the United States* (Chicago: University of Chicago Press, 1994).

2. S. Brown, *Streetwise to Sex-Wise: Sexuality Education for High-Risk Youth* (Morristown, NJ: Planned Parenthood of Greater Northern New Jersey, 1993).

3. Our Daughters & Sons: Questions and Answers for Parents of Gay, Lesbian and Bisexual People, (Washington, DC: PFLAG, 1995).

4. ACLU Fact Sheet: Overview of Lesbian and Gay Parenting, Adoption and Foster Care (New York: American Civil Liberties Union, 1999).

5. C. Patterson, Children of Lesbian and Gay Parents, *Child Development* 1025—1039 (1992).

6. American Academy of Pediatrics, Policy Statement: Homosexuality and Adolescence (RE9332), *Pediatrics* 92:4, 631—634 (October 1993).

7. F.M. Mondimore, *A Natural History of Homosexuality* (Baltimore: Johns Hopkins University, 1996).

8. A.C. Kinsey, et al., *Sexual Behavior in the Human Male* (Philadelphia: W.B. Saunders, 1948).

9. American Psychological Association, "Answers to Your Questions About Sexual Orientation and Homosexuality" (Washington, DC: American Psychological Association, July 1998).

10. Some information in this section is from "Just the Facts About Sexual Orientation & Youth: A Primer for Principals, Educators & School Personnel" (1999), a publication developed and endorsed by the American Academy of Pediatrics (AAP), American Association of School Administrators (AASA), American Counseling Association (ACA), American Federation of Teachers (AFT), American Psychological Association (APA), American School Health Association (ASHA), The Interfaith Alliance Foundation (TIAF), National Association of School Psychologists (NASP), National Association of Social Workers (NASW), and National Education Association (NEA). It is available at many Web sites, including: *www.apa.org/pi/lgbc/publications/justthefacts.html*.

11. American Academy of Pediatrics, "Policy Statement: Homosexuality and Adolescence" (RE9332), *Pediatrics* 92:4, 631–634 (October 1993).

12. "Just the Facts About Sexual Orientation & Youth: A Primer for Principals, Educators & School Personnel" (1999), a publication endorsed by the American Academy of Pediatrics (AAP), et al., p. 5.

13. "Throwaway Teens," ABC News, *20/20*, September 13, 1999.

14. K. Carter, "Gay Slurs Abound," *The Des Moines Register* (March 7, 1997).

15. S.T. Russell and K. Joyner, "Adolescent Sexual Orientation and Suicide Risk: Evidence from a National Study," *American Journal of Public Health* 91:8, 1276–1281 (2001).

16. OutProud/Oasis Internet Survey of Queer and Questioning Youth: 2000 Survey Results Preview. Found at: *www.outproud.org/survey/highlights.html*.

17. C. Ryan and D. Futterman, "Lesbian and Gay Youth: Care and Counseling," *Adolescent Medicine, State of the Art Reviews* 8:2 (June 1997).

Issue 4: Sexual Expression

1. *Sex and America's Teenagers* (New York: The Alan Guttmacher Institute, 1994).

2. M.A. Schuster, et al., "The Sexual Practices of Adolescent Virgins: Genital Sexual Activities of High School Students Who Have Never Had Intercourse," *American Journal of Public Health* 86:11,1570–1576 (1996).

3. Ibid.

4. P.F. Horan, et al., "The Meaning of Abstinence for College Students," *Journal of HIV/AIDS Prevention & Education for Adolescents and Children* 2:2, 51–66 (1998).

5. News release, *seventeen* News, "National Survey Conducted by *seventeen* Finds That More Than Half of Teens Ages 15–19 Have Engaged in Oral Sex," (February 28, 2000).

6. C. Birnbaum, "The Love & Sex Survey 2000," *Twist* 54–56 (October/November 2000).

7. H. Leitenberg, et al., "Gender Differences in Masturbation and the Relation of Masturbation Experience in Preadolescence and/or Early Adolescence to Sexual Behavior and Sexual Adjustment in Young Adulthood," *Archives of Sexual Behavior* 22:2, 87–98 (1993); and J.M. Schwartz, "Sexual Activity Prior to Coital Initiation: A Comparison Between Males and Females," *Archives of Sexual Behavior* 28:1, 63–69 (1999).

8. H. Leitenberg, et al., "Gender Differences in Masturbation and the Relation of Masturbation Experience in Preadolescence and/or Early Adolescence to Sexual Behavior and Sexual Adjustment in Young Adulthood," *Archives of Sexual Behavior* 22:2, 87–98 (1993).

9. D.F. Hurlbert and K.E. Whittaker, "The Role of Masturbation in Marital and Sexual Satisfaction: A Comparative Study of Female Masturbators and Nonmasturbators," *Journal of Sex Education and Therapy* 17:4, 272–282 (1991).

10. L. Franks, The Sex Lives of Your Children, *Talk* magazine 102—107, 157 (February 2000).

11. Reported in L. Remez, Oral Sex Among Adolescents: Is It Sex or Is It Abstinence? *Family Planning Perspectives* 32:6, 298—304 (November/December 2000).

12. Ibid.

13. For example, the Centers for Disease Control notes that Plastic food wrap can be used as a barrier *(www.cdc.gov/hiv/pubs/faq/faq19.htm)*. According to the AIDS Education Global Information System (AEGIS), Contrary to community rumors, either the microwaveable or nonmicrowaveable versions of plastic wrap can be used *(www.aegis.com/pubs/bala/1992/BA920214.html)*. Many university health services recommend using plastic wrap during oral sex.

Issue 5: Safer Sex

1. American Social Health Association, Teenagers Know More Than Adults About STDs, but Knowledge Among Both Groups Is Low, *STD News* 3:Winter, 1, 5 (1996).

2. Facts in Brief: Teen Sex and Pregnancy (New York: The Alan Guttmacher Institute, September 1999).

3. Ibid.

4. Ibid.

5. Ibid.

6. R. Bunnell, et al., High Prevalence and Incidence of Sexually Transmitted Diseases in Urban Adolescent Females Despite Moderate Risk Behaviors, *The Journal of Infectious Diseases* 180, 1624—1631 (1999).

7. J.J. Frost and J.D. Forrest, Understanding the Impact of Effective Teenage Pregnancy Prevention Programs, *Family Planning Perspectives* 27:5, 188—96 (1995); D. Kirby, et al., School-Based Programs to Reduce Sexual Risk Behaviors: A Review of Effectiveness, *Public Health Reports* 190:3, 339—60 (1994).

8. Decision Making, a publication of the SexSmarts public information partnership between the Kaiser Family Foundation and *seventeen* magazine (September 2000).

9. P. Donovan, *Testing Positive: Sexually Transmitted Disease and the Public Health Response* (New York: The Alan Guttmacher Institute, 1993).

10. Sexually Transmitted Disease, a publication of the SexSmarts public information partnership between the Kaiser Family Foundation and *seventeen* magazine (August 2001).

11. Tracking the Hidden Epidemics 2000: Trends in STDs in the United States (Atlanta, GA: Centers for Disease Control and Prevention, 2000).

12. National Institute of Allergy and Infectious Diseases, Fact Sheet: An Introduction to Sexually Transmitted Diseases (Bethesda, MD: National Institutes of Health, July 1999).

13. H.G. Miller, et al., Correlates of Sexually Transmitted Bacterial Infections Among U.S. Women in 1995, *Family Planning Perspectives* 31:1, 4—8 (1999).

14. Sexually Transmitted Disease Surveillance, 1995 (Atlanta, GA: Centers for Disease Control, 1996).

15. Department of Health and Human Services, Division of STD Prevention, Chlamydia Prevalence Monitoring Project, Sexually Transmitted Disease Surveillance 1999 Supplement, (Atlanta, GA: Centers for Disease Control and Prevention, November 2000).

16. National Center for HIV, STD and TB Prevention, Division of Sexually Transmitted Diseases, Chlamydia Disease Information (Atlanta, GA: Centers for Disease Control and Prevention, May 2001).

17. *JAMA* Patient Page: The Silent Disease, *Journal of the American Medical Association* 280:6, 582 (August 12, 1998).

18. Ibid.

19. "A Fact Sheet on Sexually Transmitted Diseases" (Menlo Park, CA: Kaiser Family Foundation, 1998).

20. C. Gorman, "Teen Girls Beware: Chlamydia Can Rob You of the Ability to Ever Have Children," *Time* magazine, 152:8 (August 24, 1998).

21. National Center for HIV, STD and TB Prevention, Division of Sexually Transmitted Diseases, "Chlamydia Disease Information" (Atlanta, GA: Centers for Disease Control and Prevention, May 2001).

22. National Institute of Allergy and Infectious Diseases, "Fact Sheet: Pelvic Inflammatory Disease" (Bethesda, MD: National Institutes of Health, July 1998).

23. National Center for HIV, STD and TB Prevention, Division of Sexually Transmitted Diseases, "Pelvic Inflammatory Disease (PID)" (Atlanta, GA: Centers for Disease Control and Prevention, May 2001).

24. Ibid.

25. Ibid.

26. National Institute of Allergy and Infectious Diseases, "Fact Sheet: Pelvic Inflammatory Disease" (Bethesda, MD: National Institutes of Health, July 1998).

27. Ibid.

28. National Center for HIV, STD and TB Prevention, Division of Sexually Transmitted Diseases, "Pelvic Inflammatory Disease (PID)" (Atlanta, GA: Centers for Disease Control and Prevention, May 2001).

29. National Institute of Allergy and Infectious Diseases, "Vaginitis Due to Vaginal Infections" (Bethesda, MD: National Institutes of Health, June 1998).

30. "A Fact Sheet on Sexually Transmitted Diseases" (Menlo Park, CA: Kaiser Family Foundation, 1998).

31. National Herpes Resource Center, "Herpes: Get the Facts" (Research Triangle Park, NC: American Social Health Association, 2001).

32. Ibid.

33. J. Trimble, et al., "Characterization of the Tumor-Associated 38-kd Protein of Herpes Simplex Virus Type II," *Journal of Reproductive Medicine* 31, supplement l, 399–409 (1986).

34. National Institute of Allergy and Infectious Diseases, "Fact Sheet: Genital Herpes" (Bethesda, MD: National Institutes of Health, March 2001).

35. M.L. Gillison, et al. "Evidence for a Causal Association Between Human Papillomavirus and a Subset of Head and Neck Cancers." *Journal of the National Cancer Institute* 92:9, 709–720, (2000).

36. L. Marr, *Sexually Transmitted Diseases: A Physician Tells You What You Need to Know* (Baltimore, MD: Johns Hopkins University Press, 1998).

37. "Tracking the Hidden Epidemics 2000: Trends in STDs in the United States" (Atlanta, GA: Centers for Disease Control and Prevention, 2000).

38. Ibid.

39. Kaiser Family Foundation/MTV/*Teen People*, "What Teens Know and Don't (But Should) About Sexually Transmitted Diseases: A National Survey of 15- to 17-year-olds" (Menlo Park, CA: Kaiser Family Foundation, 1999).

40. "Viral Hepatitis A Fact Sheet" (Atlanta, GA: Centers for Disease Control and Prevention, 2001).

41. "Viral Hepatitis B Fact Sheet" (Atlanta, GA: Centers for Disease Control and Prevention, 2001).

42. "If You Have Chronic Hepatitis B . . . " (Atlanta: GA: Centers for Disease Control and Prevention).

43. Joint United Nations Programme on HIV/AIDS (UNAIDS), "AIDS Epidemic Update: December 2000" (Geneva, Switzerland: World Health Organization, 2000).

44. "HIV and AIDS—United States, 1981–2001," *CDC/MMWR Surveillance Summaries* 50:21, 430–444 (June 2001); *HIV Prevention Strategic Plan Through 2005* (Atlanta, GA: Centers for Disease Control and Prevention, January 2001).

45. "Young People at Risk for HIV Infection" (Atlanta, GA: Centers for Disease Control and Prevention, 1999).

46. National Center for HIV, STD and TB Prevention, "Comprehensive HIV Prevention Messages for Young People (CDC Update)" (Atlanta, GA: Centers for Disease Control and Prevention, January 1997).

47. "Fact Sheet: Sexually Transmitted Diseases in the United States" (Menlo Park, CA: Kaiser Family Foundation, February 2000).

48. "Young People at Risk: HIV/AIDS Among America's Youth" (Atlanta, GA: Centers for Disease Control and Prevention, September 2000).

49. "Sexually Transmitted Diseases," a publication of the SexSmarts public information partnership between the Kaiser Family Foundation and *seventeen* magazine (August 2001).

50. Kaiser Family Foundation/MTV/*Teen People*, "What Teens Know and Don't (But Should) About Sexually Transmitted Diseases: A National Survey of 15- to 17-year-olds" (Menlo Park, CA: Kaiser Family Foundation, 1999).

51. An April 3, 1997, "NIAID News" bulletin (National Institute of Allergy and Infectious Diseases, National Institutes of Health) noted that: "Previous studies in small numbers of women suggested that N-9 [nonoxynol-9] had some benefit as a topical microbicide, but also prompted some concern that frequent use or use of high doses of N-9 could disrupt the cells that line the genital tract, thereby increasing the chances of HIV infection." An August 4, 2000, letter from Helene D. Gayle, M.D., M.P.H., the Director of the National Center for HIV, STD and TB Prevention at the Centers for Disease Control and Prevention, reported the results of a study about HIV prevention in women conducted at several locations in Africa. "At the end of the trial," Gayle wrote, "researchers found that the women who used N-9 gel had become infected with HIV at about a 50 percent higher rate than women who used the placebo gel. Further, the more frequently women used only N-9 gel (without a condom) to protect themselves, the higher their risk of becoming infected. Simply stated, N-9 did not protect against HIV infection and may have caused more transmission. Women who used N-9 also had more vaginal lesions, which might have facilitated HIV transmission . . . . [Given] that N-9 has now been proven ineffective against HIV transmission, the possibility of risk, with no benefit, indicates that N-9 should not be recommended as an effective means of HIV prevention."

52. R.F. Carey, et al., "Effectiveness of Latex Condoms as a Barrier to Human Immunodeficiency Virus-sized Particles Under the Conditions of Simulated Use," *Sexually Transmitted Diseases* 19:4, 230 (July/August 1992).

53. J. Trussell, et al., "Contraceptive Failure in the United States: An Update," *Studies in Family Planning* 21:1, 52 (January/February 1990); P. Kestelman and J. Trussell, "Efficacy of the Simultaneous Use of Condoms and Spermicides," *Family Planning Perspectives* 23:5, 227 (September/October 1991).

54. R.A. Hatcher, et al., *Contraceptive Technology*, 16th rev. ed. (New York: Irvington Publishers, Inc., 1994).

55. "Basic Facts About Condoms and Their Use in Preventing HIV Infection and Other STDs" (Atlanta, GA: Centers for Disease Control and Prevention, July 1993).

56. "Facts About Birth Control" (New York: Planned Parenthood Federation of America, 1999).

57. "Safer Sex, Condoms and 'the Pill,'" a publication of the SexSmarts public information partnership between the Kaiser Family Foundation and *seventeen* magazine (November 2000).

58. A. Glasier and D. Baird, "The Effects of Self-Administering Emergency Contraception," *The New England Journal of Medicine* 339:1, 1-4 (1998); P.F.A. Van Look and F. Stewart, "Emergency Contraception." In *Contraceptive Technology*, 17th ed., edited by R.A. Hatcher, et al., 277–295 (New York: Ardent Media, 1998).

59. Food and Drug Administration (FDA), "Prescription Drug Products; Certain Combined Oral Contraceptives for Use as Postcoital Emergency Contraception," *Federal Register* 62:37, 8609–8612 (1997).

60. Task Force on Postovulatory Methods of Fertility Regulation, "Randomised Controlled Trial of Levonorgestrel Versus the Yuzpe Regimen of Combined Oral Contraceptives for Emergency Contraception," *The Lancet* 352:9126, 428–433 (1998).

61. P.F.A. Van Look and F. Stewart, "Emergency Contraception." In *Contraceptive Technology*, 17th ed., edited by R.A. Hatcher, et al., 277–295 (New York: Ardent Media, 1998).

62. Ibid.

63. Task Force on Postovulatory Methods of Fertility Regulation, "Randomised Controlled Trial of Levonorgestrel Versus the Yuzpe Regimen of Combined Oral Contraceptives for Emergency Contraception," *The Lancet* 352:9126, 428–433 (1998); "FDA Approves Progestin-Only Emergency Contraception," *The Contraception Report* 10:5, 8–10, 16 (1999).

64. P.F.A. Van Look and F. Stewart, "Emergency Contraception." In *Contraceptive Technology*, 17th ed., edited by R.A. Hatcher, et al., 277–295 (New York: Ardent Media, 1998).

65. H. Fu, et al., "Measuring the Extent of Abortion Underreporting in the 1995 National Survey of Family Growth," *Family Planning Perspectives* 30:3 128–133 (1998); S.K. Henshaw, "Abortion Incidence and Services in the United States, 1995–1996," *Family Planning Perspectives* 30:6, 263–270, 287 (1998).

66. "Choosing Abortion—Questions and Answers" (New York: Planned Parenthood Federation of America, 1999).

67. Food and Drug Administration, Center for Drug Evaluation and Research, "Mifepristone Medication Guide" (Rockville, MD: U.S. Department of Health and Human Services, March 2001).

68. World Health Organization (WHO), Task Force on Postovulatory Methods of Fertility Regulation, "Comparison of Three Single Doses of Mifepristone as Emergency Contraception: A Randomised Trial," *The Lancet* 353, 697–702 (1999).

69. W.R. Ewart and B. Winikoff, "Toward Safe and Effective Medical Abortion," *Science* 281, 520–522 (1998).

70. C. Joffe, "Reactions to Medical Abortion Among Providers of Surgical Abortion: An Early Snapshot," *Family Planning Perspectives* 31:1, 35–38 (1999); E.A. Schaff, "Low-dose Mifepristone 200mg and Vaginal Mifepristol for Abortion" *Contraception* 59:1, 1–6 (1999).

Issue 6: Sexual Pleasure

1. E.O. Laumann, et al., *The Social Organization of Sexuality: Sexual Practices in the United States* (Chicago: University of Chicago, 1994).

2. J.K. Davidson and L.E. Hoffman, "Sexual Fantasies and Sexual Satisfaction: An Empirical Analysis of Erotic Thought," *Journal of Sex Research* 22, 184–205 (1986).

3. *Sex Education in America: A View from Inside the Nation's Classrooms* (Menlo Park, CA: Kaiser Family Foundation, September 2000).

4. National Guidelines Task Force, *Guidelines for Comprehensive Sexuality Education, Kindergarten–12th Grade*, 2nd ed. (New York: Sexuality Information and Education Council of the United States [SIECUS], 1996).

5. W. Masters and V.E. Johnson, *Human Sexual Response* (Boston: Little, Brown, 1966).

RESOURCES

General Information

BOOKS

Changing Bodies, Changing Lives: A Book for Teens on Sex and Relationships, 3rd ed., by Ruth Bell and the Teen Book Project (New York: Times Books, 1998). For ages 14–19. Thorough and nonjudgmental information on sexuality and a wide range of emotional and physical issues affecting teens, including: general emotional and physical health care, sexual harassment and violence, STIs, pregnancy, eating disorders, and positive role-modeling.

Did the Sun Shine Before You Were Born? A Sex Education Primer by Sol Gordon and Judith Gordon (Amherst, NY: Prometheus Books, 1992). For ages 4–8. Using simple language, explains how babies are created, grow in the womb, and are born. Families of various sizes and races are illustrated.

Dr. Ruth Talks to Kids: Where You Came From, How Your Body Changes, and What Sex is All About by Ruth Westheimer (New York: Aladdin Paperbacks, 1998). For preteens. Forthright exploration of the physical and emotional changes that occur during adolescence; also provides counsel on homosexuality, contraception, and STIs.

Flight of the Stork: What Children Think (and When) About Sex and Family Building, rev. ed., by Anne Bernstein (Indianapolis, IN: Perspectives Press, 1996). Designed to help parents talk to children ages 3–12 about a variety of issues including sex, adoption, infertility, surrogacy, and collaborative families.

Girls Are Girls and Boys Are Boys, So What's the Difference? A Nonsexist Sexuality Education Book for Children Ages 6 to 10 by Sol Gordon (Buffalo, NY: Prometheus Books, 1991). Information on human reproduction and the physical differences between boys and girls. In its discussion of gender, the book emphasizes that physical differences have no bearing on a person's career choice or other interests.

The "Go Ask Alice" Book of Answers: A Guide to Good Physical, Sexual, and Emotional Health by Columbia University's Health Education Program (New York: Henry Holt and Company, Inc., 1998). For teens and adults. Straightforward, nonjudgmental, and detailed answers to often difficult and embarrassing questions about physical, sexual, and emotional health. In a Q-and-A format; has a thorough resource list.

Love and Limerence: The Experience of Being in Love, 2nd ed., by Dorothy Tennov (Lantham, MD: Scarborough House, 1999). Addresses the nature of love versus the experience of infatuation and obsession, and uses the concept of limerence to explain the difference.

Period: A Girl's Guide to Menstruation with a Parent's Guide by JoAnn Loulan and Bonnie Worthern (Minnetonka, MN: Book Peddlers, 2001). For preteens. Discusses menstruation and puberty, emphasizing the importance of girls being comfortable with their bodies. Diagrams and a Q-and-A format make information easy to find and understand.

The Sex Lives of Teenagers: Revealing the Secret World of Adolescent Boys and Girls by Lynn E. Ponton (New York: Penguin Group, 2000). Uses the voices of real teens to explore their world and views on sex. Intended to help parents and teens establish better communication about adolescence and sexuality.

Sex Smart: 501 Reasons to Hold Off on Sex by Susan Browning Pogany (Minneapolis: Fairview Press, 1998). For teens. Promotes abstinence in teens, even those who have been previously sexually active. Pragmatic rather than religious in focus.

So That's How I Was Born! by Robert Brooks (New York: Aladdin Paperbacks, 1983). For ages 3–6. The book provides young children with information about human reproduction, emphasizing that shared love is the basis for conceiving a child. Includes diagrams of the human body and explanations of the differences between males and females.

The Underground Guide to Teenage Sexuality by Michael J. Basso (Minneapolis: Fairview Press, 1997). For teens. Comprehensive guide for navigating current sexuality issues which treats teens with honesty and respect while providing them with information about their bodies, relationships, and STIs.

When Sex Is the Subject: Attitudes and Answers for Young Children by Pamela M. Wilson (Santa Cruz, CA: Network Publications, 1991). Provides information on sexual development, sexuality education, and a five-step technique for answering young children's questions about sexuality.

ORGANIZATIONS

Advocates for Youth
2000 M Street NW, Suite 750
Washington, DC 20036
(202) 419-3420
www.advocatesforyouth.org
Advocates For Youth is an organization dedicated to creating and advocating programs and policies to help young people make informed and responsible choices about their reproductive and sexual health.

Alan Guttmacher Institute
120 Wall Street, 21st Floor
New York, NY 10005
(212) 248-1111
www.agi-usa.org
The Alan Guttmacher Institute (AGI) is a nonprofit organization focused on sexual and reproductive health research, policy analysis, and public education. An excellent resource for information on all aspects of sexuality and sexual health; including fact sheets, statistics, white papers, and a section on youth issues.

American Association of Sex Educators, Counselors, and Therapists (AASECT)
P.O. Box 5488
Richmond, VA 23220
www.aasect.org
A nonprofit organization, ASSECT is an association of sex educators, counselors and therapists, and professionals dedicated to promoting understanding of human sexuality and healthy sexual behavior. For a referral list of sex counselors and therapists by state, send a self-addressed stamped envelope or visit the AASECT Web site.

The Henry J. Kaiser Family Foundation
2400 Sand Hill Road
Menlo Park, CA 94025
(650) 854-9400
www.kff.org
The Henry J. Kaiser Family Foundation is an independent philanthropy focusing on the major health care issues facing the nation. The Foundation is an independent voice and source of facts and analysis for policymakers, the media, the health care community, and the general public.

National Eating Disorders Association
603 Stewart Street, Suite 803
Seattle, WA 98101
1-800-931-2237
www.nationaleatingdisorders.org
The National Eating Disorders Association is the largest nonprofit organization pledged solely to the prevention and awareness of eating disorders. It is dedicated to the elimination of eating disorders and body dissatisfaction through prevention efforts, education, referral and support services, advocacy, training, and research.

Not Me, Not Now
40 Wildbriar Road
Rochester, NY 14623
1-877-603-7306
www.notmenotnow.org
Based in Rochester, NY, Now Me, Not Now focuses on proactive pregnancy prevention with peer outreach abstinence education. It also provides advice to parents on discussing sex and strengthening communication skills.

Planned Parenthood Federation of America
434 West 33rd Street
New York, NY 10001
1-800-230-PLAN (1-800-230-7526)
www.plannedparenthood.org
Planned Parenthood is the world's largest and oldest voluntary family planning organization and is dedicated to the principles that every individual has a fundamental right to decide when or whether to have a child, and that every child should be wanted and loved. It has women's health clinics nationwide. Planned Parenthood is also an excellent information resource and serves as a clearinghouse and library of over 20,000 items including an extensive reference collection regarding sexuality issues for people with disabilities. The Web site has fact sheets and a section for teens.

Sexuality Information and Education Council of the United States (SIECUS)
130 West 42nd Street, Suite 350
New York, NY 10036
(212) 819-9770
www.siecus.org
The Sexuality Information and Education Council of the U.S. (SIECUS) is a national, nonprofit organization that affirms that sexuality is a natural and healthy part of living. SIECUS develops, collects, and disseminates information, promotes comprehensive education about sexuality, and advocates the right of individuals to make responsible sexual choices. The Web site is a rich source of information with a section for parents and a section for teens.

WEB SITES

Advocates for Youth
www.advocatesforyouth.org
Advocates for Youth is dedicated to creating programs and advocating for policies that help young people make informed and responsible decisions about their reproductive and sexual health. Has a section on the site for teens *(www.advocatesforyouth.org/teens)*.

Birds and Bees
www.birdsandbees.org
Web site for teens with information on birth control, pregnancy, and STIs. Also discusses the options of abortion, adoption, and parenting for teens who are pregnant. Sponsored by Pro-Choice Resources.

Coalition for Positive Sexuality
www.positive.org
Excellent sex information site for teens. Very down-to-earth in tone and thorough, this site for teens answers many questions about sex and offers information (in English and Spanish) about safer sex and contraception. Also offers a discussion board where teens can learn with and consult one another about sexuality issues.

Go Ask Alice!
www.goaskalice.columbia.edu
Columbia University's Go Ask Alice! provides factual, in-depth, straightforward, and nonjudgmental information in a Q-and-A format about sexuality, sexual health issues, and relationships. The site also addresses emotional and general health issues.

It's Your (Sex) Life

www.itsyoursexlife.com

The site's goal is to provide reliable and objective information about sexual health issues to young adults. Focuses on communication, HIV and STDs, pregnancy, and contraception. Sponsored by the Kaiser Family Foundation.

Iwannaknow

www.iwannaknow.org

Purpose of the site is to provide a safe, educational, and fun place for teens to learn about sexually transmitted diseases (STDs) and sexual health. Also contains a parent's guide. Sponsored by ASHA (American Social Health Association).

Scarleteen

www.scarleteen.com

Sex and sexuality resource for teen women. Provides educational information on all aspects of positive sexuality, including birth control, safe sex and sexually transmitted diseases, masturbation, anatomy, sexual orientation, sexual and romantic relationship and communication tools, abstinence, and sex.

SEX, ETC.

www.sexetc.org

A Web site by teens for teens. A place in cyberspace where teens can get accurate, up-front information about their sexuality as well as a place to get their questions answered. Topics addressed include pregnancy, STIs, sexual orientation, masturbation, abortion, sex education in schools, virginity, and date rape. Operated by the Network for Family Life Education and Rutgers University.

Talking with Kids About Tough Issues

www.talkingwithkids.org

Designed to help parents talk to their children and teens about difficult issues. Includes sections on talking about sex and about HIV and AIDS, and a list of 10 tips for talking to kids about difficult issues. Sponsored by Children Now and the Kaiser Family Foundation.

Teen Advice Online

www.teenadviceonline.org

A site by and for teens that provides information on a wide range of teen problems and issues using a network of peer advisors from around the world. Topics covered: body image, depression, teen suicide, drugs, sexual abuse, self-mutilation, pregnancy, friends, and family relationships Also has a parents' section.

Teenwire

www.teenwire.com

Sexuality, sexual health, and relationship information for teens in a site created and presented by Planned Parenthood. Includes frank but teen-friendly discussions about sex, alcohol, contraception, pregnancy, STIs, sexual assault, and abortion. Also a version of the site in Spanish.

Alcohol and Drugs

ORGANIZATIONS

Al-Anon/Alateen
1600 Corporate Landing Parkway
Virginia Beach, VA 23454-5617
1-888-4AL-ANON (1-888-425-2666)
www.al-anon.alateen.org
Al-Anon's mission is to help families and friends of alcoholics recover from the effects of living with the problem drinking of a relative or friend. Alateen, is a recovery program for young people. Alateen groups are sponsored by Al-Anon members. The recovery program is adapted from Alcoholics Anonymous and is based upon the Twelve Steps, Twelve Traditions, and Twelve Concepts of Service.

Narcotics Anonymous
P.O. Box 9999
Van Nuys, CA 91409
(818) 773-9999
www.na.org
Narcotics Anonymous provides a recovery process and support network for recovering drug addicts who are in the process of overcoming an active addiction or who are maintaining drug-free lives. The Web site has an extensive list of links to chapters and help lines worldwide.

The National Clearinghouse for Alcohol and Drug Information
P.O. Box 2345
Rockville, MD 20847-2345
1-800-729-6686
www.health.org
NCADI is the information service of the Center for Substance Abuse Prevention in the U.S. Department of Health & Human Services. NCADI is the world's largest resource for current information and materials concerning substance abuse. The Web site has sections for parents, teens, and kids. NCADI also has trained information specialists who can answer your questions 24 hours a day.

Crisis Hotlines

Childhelp USA National Child Abuse Hotline: 1-800-4-A-CHILD (1-800-422-4453)
If you suspect child abuse or need help, call the Childhelp USA National Child Abuse Hotline. The hotline is staffed 24 hours a day, 7 days a week with professional crisis counselors. Anyone can call: abused children, troubled parents, individuals concerned that abuse is occurring, and others requesting child abuse information.

The Covenant House Nineline: 1-800-999-9999
The Covenant House Nineline provides immediate crisis intervention, support, and referrals for runaways, abandoned youth, and those who are suicidal or in crisis. Help is available for children, teens, and adults.

The Girls and Boys Town National Hotline: 1-800-448-3000
The Girls and Boys Town National Hotline is a crisis hotline teens can call 24 hours a day. A professional counselor will listen and offer advice on any issue (depression, suicide, identity struggles, family troubles, and other problems).

National Runaway Switchboard: 1-800-621-4000
This toll-free number is the 24-hour hotline of the National Runaway Switchboard, a not-for-profit volunteer organization whose mission is to provide confidential crisis intervention and referrals to youth and their families. They deal with all kinds of adolescent problems, including teen depression and suicide. They can help you or your teen connect with counseling services in your area.

Depression

BOOKS

Overcoming Teen Depression: A Guide for Parents by Miriam Kaufman (Buffalo, NY: Firefly Books, 2001). Explains teen depression, incorporating up-to-date research and case studies. Discusses the warning signs, diagnosis, finding help, and current treatment approaches, including therapy, medication, and alternative treatments.

When Nothing Matters Anymore: A Survival Guide for Depressed Teens by Bev Cobain (Minneapolis: Free Spirit Publishing, 1998). Discusses the causes and types of depression, the various treatments available, and how to become and stay healthy. With true stories from teens who have dealt with depression and a discussion of depression where gender and sexuality differences are involved.

HOTLINES

The National Hopeline Network: 1-800-SUICIDE (1-800-784-2433)
The National Hopeline Network is for people who are depressed or suicidal, or those who are concerned about someone they love. It connects callers automatically to the nearest certified Crisis Center, where trained counselors answer calls 24 hours a day, 7 days a week. The Network uses the ANI (Automatic Number Identification) system to route calls. If the nearest Crisis Center is at maximum volume, the call is immediately rerouted to the next closest center. People in crisis usually reach a trained counselor within two to three rings, or about 20 to 30 seconds, from the moment they dial 1-800-SUICIDE. Callers should never encounter a busy signal or voicemail.

ORGANIZATIONS

SAVE Suicide Awareness Voices of Education
7317 Cahill Road, Suite 207
Minneapolis, MN 55439-2080
(952) 946-7998
www.save.org
Suicide Awareness Voices of Education (SAVE) is an organization dedicated to educating the public about suicide prevention and depression.

Disabilities

BOOKS

Sexuality: Your Sons and Daughters with Intellectual Disabilities by Karin Melberg Schwier and Dave Hingsburger (Baltimore: Paul H. Brookes Publishing, 2000). Helps parents help their intellectually disabled child develop a healthy and safe sexuality. Covers self-esteem, appropriate behavior, boundaries, abuse, general sexuality issues, and relationships.

ORGANIZATIONS

The Arc of the United States
1010 Wayne Avenue, Suite 650
Silver Spring, MD 20910
(301) 565-3842
www.thearclink.org
The Arc is a national organization on mental retardation with state and local chapters throughout the United States. Several sexuality-related publications are available from The Arc including *The Sexuality Policy and Procedure Manual.*

National Information Center for Children and Youth with Disabilities (NICHCY)
P.O. Box 1492
Washington, DC 20013
1-800-695-0285
www.nichcy.org
NICHCY is a national information clearinghouse with a special focus on children and youth (birth to age 22) with disabilities. *Sexuality Education for Children and Youth with Disabilities,* which deals with education related to the social-sexual development of youth with disabilities, was published for parents and professionals as part of their *News Digest* series.

Pregnancy

ORGANIZATIONS

Birthright International
777 Coxwell Avenue
Toronto, Ontario, M4C 3C6
Canada
1-800-550-4900
www.birthright.org
Birthright is a nonprofit organization that provides nonjudgmental support to girls and women who are faced with an unplanned pregnancy. It counsels about abortion alternatives. All services are free, confidential, and available to any woman regardless of age, race, creed, economic or marital status.

The National Abortion Federation
1755 Massachusetts Avenue NW, Suite 600
Washington, DC 20036
1-800-772-9100
www.prochoice.org
The National Abortion Federation is a resource organization for those who find themselves with an unwanted or unexpected pregnancy and want to understand their options before making a decision. The organization provides confidentiality, information on pregnancy and abortion, and local referrals.

National Campaign to Prevent Teen Pregnancy
1776 Massachusetts Avenue NW, Suite 200
Washington, DC 20036
(202) 478-8500
www.teenpregnancy.org
The mission of the National Campaign to Prevent Teen Pregnancy is to improve the well-being of children, youth, and families by reducing teen pregnancy. Site has useful information for parents and a section for teens. Has a wide variety of fact sheets, statistics, tips, and resources available on the site and from the organization.

Safer Sex

BOOKS

All About Birth Control: A Personal Guide by John Knowles and Marcia Ringel (New York: Three Rivers Press, 1998). Comprehensively documents most contraceptive choices available in the United States. Discusses pros and cons of each type of contraception; includes a chapter to help people choose the contraception right for them.

The Complete Guide to Safer Sex, rev. ed., by The Institute for Advanced Study of Human Sexuality (New York: Barricade Books, 1999). Takes a practical, comprehensive, and sex-positive approach to discussing the prevention of AIDS and other STIs. Relies on both clinical and plainspoken language at various points in the text.

Contraception: A Guide to Birth Control Methods, 2nd ed., by Vern Bullough and Bonnie Bullough (Amherst, NY: Prometheus Books, 1997). A comprehensive work presenting detailed information on most birth control options currently available, rating them on success rates, safety, medical and psychological affects, and legality. Also includes an historical overview of contraception and the latest research into new birth control methods.

Sexually Transmitted Diseases: A Physician Tells You What You Need to Know (A Johns Hopkins Press Health Book) by Lisa Marr, M.D. (Baltimore, MD: Johns Hopkins University Press, 1999). Up-to-date material on 22 different STDs, detailing the prevalence, symptoms, transmittal, diagnoses, and treatments of each; also covers anatomy and safer sex.

HOTLINES

CDC Hepatitis Hotline: 1-888-4-HEP-CDC (1-888-443-7232)
A service of the CDC s Division of Viral Hepatitis, this 24-hour hotline provides recorded information and fact sheets by fax. There is also an option to speak to a live counselor about viral hepatitis issues.

CDC National AIDS Hotline: 1-800-342-AIDS (1-800-342-2437)
The National AIDS Hotline is the world s largest health information service. It operates 24 hours a day, 7 days a week. Trained information specialists answer questions about HIV infection and AIDS and provide referrals to appropriate services including clinics, hospitals, local hotlines, counseling and testing sites, legal services, health departments, support groups, educational organizations, and service agencies throughout the United States.

CDC National STD Hotline: 1-800-227-8922 or 1-800-342-2437
A service of the CDC s National Center for HIV, STD and TB Prevention, Division of Sexually Transmitted Diseases, the National STD Hotline provides anonymous, confidential information on sexually transmitted diseases (STDs) and how to prevent them. It also provides referrals to clinical and other services. Operates 24 hours a day, 7 days a week.

Emergency Contraception Hotline: 1-888-NOT-2-LATE (1-888-668-2528)
Operated by the Princeton Office of Population Research in New Jersey and the Reproductive Health Technologies Project in Washington, D.C., this 24-hour hotline provides the names and numbers of clinicians in a caller s geographic area who prescribe emergency contraception.

National Herpes Hotline: (919) 361-8488
The National Herpes Hotline is operated by the American Social Health Association (ASHA) as part of the Herpes Resource Center (HRC). The hotline provides accurate information and appropriate referrals to anyone concerned about herpes. Trained specialists are available to answer questions related to transmission, prevention, and treatment. Also provides support for emotional issues surrounding herpes, such as self-esteem and partner communication. Hours: 9 A.M. to 6 P.M., EST, Monday through Friday.

National HPV and Cervical Cancer Prevention Hotline: (919) 361-4848
The National HPV and Cervical Cancer Prevention Hotline is operated by the American Social Health Association (ASHA) as part of the HPV and Cervical Cancer Prevention Resource Center. It provides current information on the virus and its link to cancer, and offers free information to the public about risk reduction, diagnosis, and treatment of HPV and the prevention of cervical cancer. Trained specialists are available to address questions related to transmission, prevention, and treatment of HPV. The hotline also provides support for emotional issues surrounding HPV, such as self-esteem and partner communication. Hours: 1 P.M. to 6 P.M., EST, Monday through Friday.

Planned Parenthood Emergency Contraception Hotline: 1-800-230-PLAN (1-800-230-7526)
Call toll-free for a confidential appointment to arrange for emergency contraception at the nearest Planned Parenthood, or to schedule a pregnancy test.

ORGANIZATIONS

American Social Health Association
P.O. Box 13827
Research Triangle Park, NC 27713
www.ashastd.org
ASHA s mission is to stop sexually transmitted diseases and their harmful consequences to individuals, families, and communities. Provides information about a variety of STDs, with hotline numbers and details (see the National Herpes Hotline on page 235 and the National HPV and Cervical Cancer Prevention Hotline above).

The Centers for Disease Control and Prevention (CDC)
1600 Clifton Road
Atlanta, GA 30333
(404) 639-3534
www.cdc.gov
An excellent source of information on STDs/STIs, the CDC has the Division of Sexually Transmitted Diseases, which is rich in accurate and current information about a variety of STDs *(www.cdc.gov/nchstp/dstd/dstdp.html)*. The main CDC Web site has a very complete FAQ on HIV and AIDS, and the results of long-term studies into teen behavior.

National Institute of Allergy and Infectious Diseases (NIAID)
Office of Communication and Public Liaison
Building 31, Room 7A50-MSC #2520
Bethesda, MD 20892
(301) 496-5717
www.niaid.nih.gov
An excellent source of information on STIs *(www.niaid.nih.gov/dmid/stds)*. Has a variety of fact sheets detailing symptoms, the diagnosis process, treatments, complications, and prevention. Also a good source for statistics and the most recent news and research on STIs.

WEB SITES

Birth Control Information
www.plannedparenthood.org/bc
Offers explanations of the different forms of birth control, how effective each is, and the effect each has on the body.

Not-2-Late: The Emergency Contraception Website
ec.princeton.edu or not-2-late.com
Provides accurate information about all aspects of emergency contraception, including a detailed FAQ list, a directory of providers, and current news and research. Operated by the Office of Population Research at Princeton University. In English, Spanish, and French.

Sexual Abuse and Sexual Assault

BOOKS

How Long Does It Hurt? A Guide to Recovering from Incest and Sexual Abuse for Teenagers, Their Friends, and Their Families by Cynthia L. Mather with Kristina E. Debye (San Francisco: Jossey-Bass, 1994). Addresses the issues and emotions raised by incest and sexual abuse in a methodical, step-by-step manner. For both male and female survivors.

The Me Nobody Knows: A Guide for Teen Survivors by Barbara Bean and Shari Bennett (San Francisco: Jossey-Bass, 1997). Guide addresses the emotions raised by sexual abuse, while offering direct and practical advice on reporting the abuse and seeking counseling. Contains first-person stories by teens.

ORGANIZATIONS

Rape, Abuse & Incest National Network (RAINN)
635–B Pennsylvania Avenue SE
Washington, DC 20003
The National Sexual Assault Hotline: 1-800-656-HOPE (1-800-656-4673)
www.rainn.org
The Rape, Abuse & Incest National Network (RAINN) is a nonprofit organization based in Washington, D.C., which offers free, confidential counseling and support 24 hours a day, 7 days a week via a national crisis hotline for victims of sexual assault. It provides confidentiality, support, and the nearest local referrals for additional help. The hotline is free and confidential. When a victim calls the 800-number, the call is immediately routed to the rape crisis center nearest the caller. RAINN has more than 1,000 crisis center affiliates across America.

Sexual Orientation

BOOKS

Beyond Acceptance: Parents of Lesbians and Gays Talk About Their Experiences, rev. ed., by Carolyn Welch Griffin, et al. (New York: St. Martin's Press, 1996). Discusses the varied and common reactions, issues, and anxieties parents have when they find out about their child's sexuality. Contains first-person insights from parents and practical suggestions.

Free Your Mind: The Book for Gay, Lesbian, and Bisexual Youth—and Their Allies by Ellen Bass and Kate Kaufman (New York: HarperPerennial, 1996). Comprehensive resource with information and practical advice for GLBT youth, including: self-discovery, coming out, friends, relationships, family, school, and community.

Is It a Choice? Answers to 300 of the Most Frequently Asked Questions About Gay and Lesbian People, rev. ed., by Eric Marcus (San Francisco: Harper San Francisco, 1999). A compendium of insightful, frank, and clear answers to commonly asked questions about homosexuality.

Now That You Know: A Parents' Guide to Understanding Their Gay and Lesbian Children, 3rd ed., by Betty Fairchild and Nancy Hayward (San Diego, CA: Harcourt Brace, 1998). Explores homosexuality and the impact of the coming out process; encourages parents to be supportive of gay and lesbian children. Supplies support group information and resources.

HOTLINES

Trevor Helpline: 1-866-488-7386
This hotline offers youth support and suicide prevention services 24 hours a day, 7 days a week.

ORGANIZATIONS

Children of Lesbians and Gays Everywhere
3543 18th Street #1
San Francisco, CA 94110
(415) 861-5437
www.colage.org
Children of Lesbians and Gays Everywhere (COLAGE) is the only international organization specifically supporting young people with gay, lesbian, bisexual, or transgender parents. COLAGE fosters the growth of children through education, support from local to international levels, advocating the rights of families, and promoting acceptance in the general community.

OutProud—The National Coalition for Gay, Lesbian, Bisexual & Transgender Youth
369 Third Street, Suite B-362
San Rafael, CA 94901
www.outproud.org
OutProud serves the needs of young GLBT men and women by providing advocacy, information, resources and support. The organization's goal is to help GLBT youth become happy, successful, confident and vital gay, lesbian and bisexual adults. Services include: outreach and support, networking, and grassroots activism on issues pertaining to GLBT youth.

Parents and Friends of Lesbians and Gays (PFLAG)
1726 M Street NW, Suite 400
Washington, DC 20036
(202) 467-8180
www.pflag.org
PFLAG is a national nonprofit organization of parents, families, and friends of lesbian, gay, bisexual, and transgender individuals. Their mission is to promote the health and well-being of GLBT persons, their families, and their friends through support, education, and advocacy. It provides opportunities for dialogue about sexual orientation and gender identity, and acts to create a society that is healthy and respectful of human diversity.

GLOSSARY

abortion

the termination or ending of a pregnancy. Spontaneous abortion, also called a miscarriage, refers to a pregnancy that is lost on its own, naturally.

abstinence

the state of not being active sexually. Sometimes used to refer specifically to abstaining from sexual intercourse. Also referred to as celibacy or chastity.

acne

a condition caused by clogged and irritated pores which results in pimples, whiteheads, and blackheads.

acquaintance rape

when sexual behavior is forced upon a person by someone he or she knows and may even have had sex with willingly on previous occasions. Also known as date rape.

the Adolescent

the part of an individual's personality that develops around the time of puberty. Its goal is to separate from the family of origin and discover sexual identity and personal strengths and weaknesses. It is often competitive and insecure. Part of the Miron Model.

the Adult

the part of an individual's personality that has worked through the insecurity and power issues of childhood and the sexual identity, independence, and competition issues of adolescence. The Adult has developed its own sense of self and is not defined by other people's opinions. Some individuals may never develop the Adult aspect of their personality. Part of the Miron Model.

AIDS

acquired immune deficiency syndrome, a suppression of the body's immune system caused by the HIV virus, which leaves the body unable to fight infections. Currently, there is no cure.

anal sex

the insertion of a penis or object into the anus of another person. It is a form of pleasure for some heterosexuals as well as some homosexuals. This activity is considered a high-risk behavior for sexually transmitted infections. Sometimes called sodomy.

androgens

male sex hormones that promote secondary sex characteristics and influences sex drive. It is produced in the testes of men and the adrenal glands of both sexes.

animal skin condoms

a condom made from some part of an animal. It is thinner than latex and may protect against pregnancy but not against sexually transmitted infections.

aphrodisiac

something believed to stimulate or enhance sexual interest, although no reliable evidence exists to support the effectiveness of any aphrodisiac. Some substances believed to be aphrodisiacs may, in fact, be dangerous.

areola

the area of darkened skin surrounding the nipple of the breast.

axillary hair

hair under the arms.

bacteria

microscopic organisms that may cause disease. Antibiotics are used to fight off bacteria.

bacterial vaginosis

a common vaginal infection. The exact causes are unknown, though women who have a new sex partner or who have had many sex partners are more likely to get it.

Bartholin's glands

two small glands located at the opening of the vagina. They secrete lubricating fluids when a woman is aroused.

ben-wa balls

round balls, usually made of metal, used in pairs and inserted in the vagina. When a woman rocks back and forth, the inside of the vagina is stimulated. They should not be used for prolonged periods of time.

birth control

various ways to plan for or prevent pregnancy. Also called contraception.

birth control pills

pills containing varying amounts of the female hormones estrogen and progesterone. When taken properly, they protect a woman from pregnancy but not from sexually transmitted infections. An oral prescription method of birth control. Also called the pill.

bisexual

a person who is romantically and sexually attracted to both men and women.

breast

the fatty tissue deposited behind the nipple. Women's breasts contain glands that can produce milk during and after a pregnancy for nursing the baby.

Candida albicans

see vaginal yeast infection.

casual sex

sexual behavior engaged in without a long-term commitment to a relationship.

celibacy
the state of abstaining from sexual behavior. Also known as abstinence or chastity.

cervical cap
a thimble-shaped latex dome that fits snugly onto the cervix and is fitted internally for a woman by a health care provider. Once fitted, it is inserted by the woman as needed. Must be used with a spermicidal cream, jelly, or foam to be effective at preventing pregnancy. Offers no protection from sexually transmitted infections.

cervix
the lower portion, or neck, of the uterus.

chancre
a painless sore with a raised edge that occurs during stage 1 syphilis. It is highly infectious.

chancroid
a bacterial infection that is spread by sexual contact.

the Child
the part of an individual's personality that forms during childhood. It often feels inferior, insecure, and powerless. It is also a source of wonder and joy. Part of the Miron Model.

chlamydia
a common sexually transmitted bacterial infection that can be found alone or sometimes in conjunction with gonorrhea. Currently, it is the most common sexually transmitted infection in the United States.

cilia
little hairs that line the fallopian tubes and move the egg toward the uterus.

circumcision
the removal of the foreskin from the penis.

clitoral hood
the fold of skin that covers the clitoris.

clitoris
the most sexually sensitive part of the female body, located just above the urethral and vaginal openings. The clitoris becomes erect as a woman becomes sexually excited. For most women, stimulation of the clitoris is an important source of arousal for reaching orgasm.

cock ring
a ring placed at the base of an erect penis used to prolong erection. It can be dangerous if used for an extended period of time, because it restricts blood flow.

coitus
penile-vaginal sexual intercourse.

coitus interruptus
interrupting intercourse by withdrawing the penis from the vagina before ejaculation. This is a poor method of birth control, since sperm may be present in fluids secreted before ejaculation (pre-ejaculatory fluid). Provides no protection from sexually transmitted infections. Also called withdrawal.

coming out
the personal awareness and public acknowledgment that a person is homosexual or bisexual. This process may take a very long time to complete.

conception
the process that unites sperm and egg to form a potential new life.

condom
a sheath or covering made from various materials that is placed over an erect penis to protect from pregnancy. Condoms can be made of latex, polyurethane, or animal skins. Condoms made of latex can help prevent the contraction of sexually transmitted infections.

contraception
the prevention of conception or pregnancy. Also known as birth control.

contraceptive cream
a cream containing a spermicide that is inserted deep into the vagina prior to intercourse in order to protect against pregnancy. Offers no protection from sexually transmitted infections.

contraceptive foam
a foam containing a spermicide inserted with an applicator into the very back of the vagina, covering the cervix and protecting against pregnancy. Offers no protection from sexually transmitted infections.

contraceptive suppository
a waxy, bullet-shaped object that dissolves when it is inserted into the back of the vagina, releasing a spermicide that covers the cervix and protects against pregnancy. Offers no protection from sexually transmitted infections.

corona
the ridge or rim around the head or glans of the penis.

corpora cavernosa
two cylinder-like structures inside the penis and clitoris that can fill with blood and cause erection.

corpus spongiosum
a cylinder-like structure inside the bottom area of the penis that can fill with blood and cause erection. The urethra passes through the center of this structure.

Cowper's glands
two glands inside the man's body, located below the prostate gland. They secrete an alkaline substance (pre-ejaculatory fluid or pre-cum) that lines the urethra to neutralize any acid remaining from urine. It may contain enough sperm to cause pregnancy.

cunnilingus
oral stimulation of the female genitals.

date rape
see acquaintance rape.

dental dam
a thin latex sheet used by dentists to isolate an area in the mouth. May be used in sexual activity to cover the vulva during oral stimulation for protection against sexually transmitted infections.

Depo-Provera
a prescription method of birth control where an injection of progestin is given to a woman every twelve weeks to avoid pregnancy. Offers no protection from sexually transmitted infections. Also called depo shots or the shot.

dermatologist
a doctor who specializes in skin problems.

diaphragm
a latex dome that covers the cervix and is fitted internally for a woman by a health care provider. Once fitted, it is inserted by the woman as needed. Must be used with a spermicidal cream, jelly, or foam to be effective at preventing pregnancy. Offers no protection from sexually transmitted infections.

double standard
the belief that it's okay for men to engage in sexual behavior, but not women.

douche
the washing out of the inside of the vagina. Not recommended unless directed by a health care professional.

dysmenorrhea
problematic or painful menstruation.

ectopic pregnancy
a life-threatening condition in which the fertilized egg grows outside the uterus, usually in a fallopian tube. Ectopic pregnancy results in miscarriage and is potentially fatal for the mother. Also called tubal pregnancy.

egg
technically called an ovum (the plural is ova). A woman is born with between 100,000 and 300,000 potential eggs in each ovary.

ejaculate
the combination of fluid and sperm cells expelled from the penis during orgasm. On average, a man expels approximately one teaspoon, which contains between 200 million and 400 million sperm.

ejaculation
the act of expelling semen from the penis in a series of spurts, or spasms, that result from the contraction of various internal glands and muscles.

emergency contraception
comes in two forms. Emergency contraceptive pills are given in two doses, within 72 hours of an act of unprotected sex to insure that pregnancy does not take place. Also called morning after pills. Copper IUD insertion can be used within five days of unprotected intercourse to prevent pregnancy. Neither offers protection from sexually transmitted infections.

endometrium
the inner lining of the uterus. Under the influence of hormones, it builds up and sloughs off in rhythmic cycles known as menstruation.

epididymis
the stocking-shaped internal structure that sits on top of each testicle and serves as a storage area where sperm mature.

erection
the stiffening and enlargement of the penis, clitoris, labia minora, or nipples caused by blood trapped inside special areas of these structures. It is usually, but not exclusively, a response to sexual arousal.

erotica
sexually arousing material—books, magazines, movies, videos, audio recordings, Web sites, etc.—that is not considered offensive to the average person. It also has goals other than sexual arousal such as artistic expression.

estrogen
a female sex hormone, produced mainly in the ovaries and, to a lesser degree, in the adrenal gland. It is responsible for many changes in a woman's body at puberty and continues to affect her menstrual cycle. It is found in smaller amounts in men.

fallopian tubes
two narrow tubes connected to the top of the uterus that form a pathway for an egg to travel from the ovary to the uterus. A mature egg is encouraged into the fallopian tube by the enlarged ends of the tubes called fimbria. Conception usually takes place here.

fellatio
oral stimulation of a penis.

female condom
a polyurethane pouch with flexible rings at both ends that is inserted into the vagina. The back end covers the cervix and walls of the vagina. The vulva is covered by the open end. Helps protect against pregnancy and sexually transmitted infections.

fertilization
the penetration of the egg by a sperm, which results in conception.

foam
see contraceptive foam.

foreplay
the various forms of interaction and pleasuring between two people that increase sexual arousal and usually, but not necessarily, precede sexual intercourse.

foreskin
a fold of skin that covers the head of the penis. It may be removed by a process known as circumcision. It is also called prepuce.

French kiss
a kiss involving the placing and moving of the tongue in the partner's mouth for sexual pleasure.

frigid
an old term that means a lack of sexual responsiveness.

fun-sex
a category of sexual encounters in which the couple is interested in the fun and enjoyment of each other. Although it may take place in a loving relationship, love is not a necessary component in this flavor of sex.

gay
a widely used term for homosexual. Although it can be used for both men and women, it more frequently refers to male homosexuals.

gay rights
refers to the rights of homosexuals not to be discriminated against in areas such as employment, housing, insurance benefits, etc.

gender
whether a person is male or female.

gender identity
a person's experiences of himself or herself as male or female.

gender role
the behaviors and characteristics expected of a male or female in a particular culture. Also called sex role.

genitals
the sexual organs of men and women.

genital warts
see human papillomavirus.

glans
the tip of the clitoris or penis; also known as the head or corona.

gonads
the sex glands (ovaries and testicles) of men and women.

gonorrhea
a sexually transmitted infection caused by a bacteria. Also known as the drip or the clap. Untreated, it can lead to sterility in both men and women.

Grafenberg spot (G-spot)
a sexually sensitive area on the inside front wall of the vagina. Also called the G-spot.

the Grown-up
a person of any age who is controlled by the Adolescent or Child part of himself or herself.

gynecologist
a doctor who specializes in the care and treatment of a woman's reproductive system.

harassment
unwanted, uninvited looks, behaviors, and gestures that create a threatening environment.

hepatitis
a family of five viruses that can affect the liver. Hepatitis B (HBV) is the one most closely associated with sexual transmission, though type A can also be spread sexually. There are hepatitis A and B vaccines.

herpes
caused by the herpes simplex virus (HSV). It causes painful blisters and is spread by skin-to-skin contact with an infectious area. There is symptom relief but no known cure. Genital herpes may increase a woman's chances of developing cancer of the cervix.

heterosexual
a person who is romantically and sexually attracted to people of the other sex.

homophobia
fear of or hostility toward homosexuals (lesbians and gay men).

homosexual
a person who is romantically and sexually attracted to people of the same sex.

hormones
chemical substances secreted directly into the bloodstream that act as messengers. Estrogen, progesterone, and testosterone are among the most important hormones affecting sexuality and reproduction.

human immunodeficiency virus (HIV)
a virus spread through blood, semen, vaginal secretions, and breast milk. It attacks the body's immune system and gradually leaves the infected person unable to fight off infections and diseases. Eventually develops into AIDS, which has no known cure.

human papillomavirus (HPV)
caused by the human papillomavirus. It results in warts on the infected areas. The warts are very contagious and are spread through oral, genital, or anal sex with an infected partner. Also called HPV, genital warts, and venereal warts.

hymen
a thin membrane that partially covers the opening of the vagina of most women and girls who have not had sexual intercourse. Contains one or more holes to allow for the exit of menstrual flow.

incest
sexual activity between closely related family members.

intersexed
a person born with physical characteristics that differ from what males and females are typically expected to have, or a mixture of male and female genitalia. Also called hermaphrodite.

intrauterine device
a plastic or metal device inserted into the uterus by a health care professional to prevent pregnancy. Offers no protection from sexually transmitted infections. Commonly known as an IUD.

inverted nipple
the turning inward of the nipple.

labia majora
part of the vulva, the larger, fleshy outer lips which cover and protect the vaginal opening. They are covered with pubic hair.

labia minora
part of the vulva, the smaller, sensitive inner lips covering the vaginal opening. Made of erectile tissue, the labia minora swell and open the vaginal area when a woman is sexually excited. No pubic hair is present on these lips. They meet above the clitoris to form the clitoral hood.

larynx
a structure in the throat that contains the vocal chords and enlarges in males during puberty, causing the traditionally deeper voice of men.

lesbian
a woman who is romantically and sexually attracted to other women.

limerence
a made up word to describe the strong feelings of attraction in the early phase of a relationship, which may or may not continue throughout a relationship.

love-sex
a type of sexual encounter whose goal is to communicate the love that each partner is feeling for the other.

lubricate
to make slippery or wet. The vagina lubricates when a woman is sexually aroused.

lubricant
a substance that causes a slipperiness. Only water-based lubricants should be used in the vaginal or anal area.

Lunelle
a prescription method of birth control where an injection of estrogen and progesterone is given to a woman every month to avoid pregnancy. Offers no protection from sexually transmitted infections.

masturbation
stimulation of one's own genitals and body to provide sexual pleasure. Also known as self-pleasuring.

menarche
a woman's first menstrual cycle, or period.

menstruation
the rhythmic cycling of a woman's hormones that cause a build-up and sloughing off of the inner lining of the uterus. Also called a period.

metacommunication
focusing a conversation on the process or style of the communication rather than on the content.

mifepristone
a drug that can be used as emergency contraception. It blocks progesterone and helps prevent pregnancy. Formerly called RU-486.

miscarriage
the natural, spontaneous loss of a pregnancy. Also known as spontaneous abortion.

monogamous
having only one sexual or marital partner at a time.

mons veneris
a fatty deposit over the pubic bone of a woman, which is covered with pubic hair.

nipple
the tip of the breast which is made up of erectile tissue. In the woman, the nipple has many holes through which breast milk may pass to feed a baby.

nocturnal emission
a male's secretion of semen while sleeping. Also called a wet dream.

nongonococcal urethritis (NGU)
inflammation of the urethra caused by something other than gonorrhea. Most commonly caused by chlamydia, but can also be caused by parasites, fungi, other bacteria, or allergic reactions. Also known as nonspecific urethritis (NSU).

nonoxynol-9
the active ingredient in many spermicides.

Norplant
a series of six small rods containing synthetic progestin that are implanted inside the upper arm of a woman by a health care practitioner to prevent pregnancy. A prescription method of birth control. Norplant offers no protection from sexually transmitted infections.

obstetrician
a doctor who takes care of pregnant women, helps in the delivery of babies, and delivers post-partum care to both mothers and infants.

oral sex
sexual stimulation of the genitals by the mouth. Also called fellatio and cunnilingus.

orgasm
the pleasurable buildup and sudden release of sexual tension. Also called a climax.

outercourse
any sexual behavior that does not include oral, anal, or vaginal contact with either vaginal secretions or semen.

ovaries
the two gonads, or sex glands, of the female. They contain eggs and produce the female hormones estrogen and progesterone.

ovulation
the release of a mature ovum from the ovary.

ovum
technical term for an egg. The plural is ova.

PAP test
a common medical test that examines cervical cells to see if they are normal or abnormal (leading toward cancer or cancerous). Also called a PAP smear.

pelvic inflammatory disease (PID)
infection in the uterus and pelvic area, usually caused by a sexually transmitted infection. The most common and serious complication of sexually transmitted infections in women (aside from AIDS). Can lead to sterility and ectopic (tubal) pregnancies if left untreated. Also known as PID.

penis
the external male sexual organ which becomes erect when sexually excited. Urine or semen exit a man's body through a hole at the tip of the head.

pornography
media created strictly for the purpose of sexual arousal.

pre-ejaculatory fluid
a fluid secreted by the Cowper's glands to neutralize the acidity of the man's urethra. Men usually cannot feel when this is secreted. It may contain sperm. Also called pre-cum.

pregnancy
a state in which a growing organism develops in the uterus of its mother.

premenstrual syndrome
a cluster of physical and emotional symptoms that can occur a few days before menstruation. Also called PMS.

progesterone
a female hormone manufactured primarily in the ovaries and secondarily in the adrenal glands, whose key function is to help prepare the uterus for the possibility of pregnancy.

prophylactic
see condom.

prostaglandin
a chemical that can contract or relax a smooth muscle.

prostate gland
a chestnut-shaped gland found inside a man's body just below the bladder. The urethra (the structure that carries urine or semen) passes through it. The prostate supplies some of the fluid that makes up semen and is primarily responsible for the pressure of ejaculation.

puberty
a time in life when a person becomes sexually mature and able to reproduce.

pubic hair
the darker, curlier, coarser hair that grows on the scrotum and above the penis in men and on the labia majora and mons veneris in women.

pubic lice
tiny insects that cause a rash and intense itching in the pubic area. Most often spread through sexual contact. Also called crabs.

rape
being forced into sexual intercourse against one's will.

recreational drugs
nonprescription drugs that are taken, often illegally, for various effects. For example, marijuana, methamphetamines, cocaine, LSD, and heroin.

refractory period
a period of time after orgasm during which further sexual response is not possible for a man. The amount of time lengthens gradually with age. Not found in women.

rhythm method
a method of birth control that tracks changes in a woman's body during her menstrual cycle to identify the time when ovulation most likely occurs. Sexual intercourse is not engaged in the three to four days before and after ovulation. Offers no protection from sexually transmitted infections. Also called natural birth control.

safer sex
various behaviors that minimize the possibility of exchanging body fluids and, therefore, help protect against pregnancy and sexually transmitted infections.

scabies
tiny mites spread primarily through sexual contact that cause intense itching and red bumps.

scrotum
the sac of loose, wrinkled skin under the penis that contains a man's testicles.

secondary sex characteristics
physical characteristics of mature women and men that develop at puberty, such as body hair, breasts, deepening voice, etc.

self-pleasuring
see masturbation.

semen
a mixture of sperm and fluids from various glands which is ejaculated by a man. Also known as cum.

seminal vesicles
two glands inside the male that produce much of the fluid in semen.

sex discrimination
the inequality of treatment, commonly in the area of employment, based simply on one's sex.

sex-sex
a kind of sex engaged in for the release of sexual tension. It can exist in loving relationships, but love is not required for this type of sex.

sexual exploration games
games that many young children play with children of roughly the same age.

sexual harassment
unwanted, uninvited sexual looks, behaviors, and gestures, usually involving coercion and a difference in status or power between the people involved.

sexual intercourse
the act of putting the penis inside another person's body.

sexually transmitted infection (STI)
any one of a group of diseases, infections, and parasites that are passed from one person to another through sexual contact. Used to be called STDs (sexually transmitted diseases) and VD (venereal disease).

sexual orientation
a person's emotional and sexual attraction to people of the same sex (homosexual), the other sex (heterosexual), or both sexes (bisexual).

smegma
a white cheese-like substance that can collect under the foreskin of the penis or the clitoral hood.

sperm
the reproductive sex cell of a man that is produced in the testicles and ejaculated out of the penis in semen.

spermatic cord
a cord attached to the testicle that allows it to rise or drop in the scrotal sac.

spermicide
a chemical that kills sperm, for example, nonoxynol-9.

stereotype
an oversimplified way of viewing all members of a group.

sterility
the inability to conceive a child.

STI
see sexually transmitted infection.

syphilis
a sexually transmitted infection caused by bacteria.

testicle
the male gonad, or sex gland, that is responsible for the production of sperm and male hormones. Males have two testicles contained within the scrotum.

testosterone
the primary sex hormone of the male, mainly produced by the testicles. Also produced by the adrenal glands of both men and women. Believed to be responsible for sex drive.

toxic shock syndrome (TSS)
a serious and potentially life threatening condition caused by a bacteria. A possible contributing factor to the buildup of bacteria in the vagina may be the use of super absorbent tampons. Nothing should be left in the vagina for longer than 6–8 hours.

transgendered
a person who may have characteristics, behaviors, and self-perceptions typical of, or more commonly associated with, persons of the other sex.

transsexual
a person who feels he or she was born into a body of the wrong biological sex and seeks to do something about it, usually by hormone therapies and/or surgery.

trichomoniasis
a sexually transmitted infection caused by a protozoan parasite and results in the inflammation of the genitals. Also called trich.

tubal ligation
a method of birth control that is best considered permanent, involving the interruption of the fallopian tubes so that an egg cannot be fertilized. Offers no protection from sexually transmitted infections.

urethra
the structure that carries urine from the bladder to the outside of the body. In men, semen also passes through the urethra.

urethral bulb
part of the urethra contained within the prostate.

uterus
the organ in a woman that holds and nurtures a developing baby. When the woman is not pregnant, it discharges its lining monthly in a process called menstruation. Also known as the womb.

vagina
a flexible and muscular organ, which in a sexually nonaroused state collapses, but which can stretch to allow for sexual intercourse or the passing of a baby. Sensitive at the opening but relatively insensitive at the back.

vaginal contraceptive film
a thin sheet of material containing a spermicide. When placed properly at the cervix at the very back of the vagina, it will dissolve, covering the cervix with spermicide, and protect against pregnancy. Offers no protection from sexually transmitted infections.

vaginal contraceptive ring
a flexible ring about 2.1 inches in diameter and containing estrogen and progestin that is inserted into the vagina for three weeks of each month to prevent pregnancy. A new ring is used each month. It is a prescription method of birth control and offers no protection from sexually transmitted infections.

vaginal lubrication
the secretions of the vagina that occur when a woman becomes aroused sexually.

vaginal yeast infection
an overgrowth of a fungus (*Candida albicans*) that lives in a healthy vagina, usually without causing any problems. Can be triggered by a number of factors including antibiotics, birth control pills, douching, a change in diet, and diabetes. Also known as candidiasis.

vaginitis
inflammation of the vaginal walls which may be caused by a variety of agents, including infections, lack of estrogen, irritants, and allergies.

vas deferens
two tubes, each about 16 inches long, which carry sperm from the epididymis on top of the testicles to the base of the prostate gland.

vasectomy
a method of birth control for males that is best considered permanent. Consists of tying, cutting, or otherwise interrupting a portion of the vas deferens thus preventing sperm from becoming part of the semen. Offers no protection from sexually transmitted infections.

vasocongestion
the closing of the veins and the opening of the arteries in an area, causing blood to accumulate.

vibrator
an electrical or battery-operated device that vibrates. When applied to the area around the clitoris or penis, it can cause orgasm.

Victorian era
a time in England and other English-speaking countries when any discussions of sexuality or sensuality was taboo. Roughly mid-1800s to early 1900s.

virgin
a person who has not had sexual intercourse.

virus
an organism that invades a cell and uses the cell to create more viral material.

vulva
the external sexual organs of a woman, which include the mons veneris, labia majora, labia minora, clitoris, and openings of the urethra and vagina.

wet dream
the involuntary ejaculation of semen during sleep. Also called nocturnal emission.

withdrawal
see coitus interruptus.

womb
another term for the uterus.

INDEX

ABOUT THE AUTHORS

Amy and Charles Miron, a Baltimore-based husband-and-wife team, are sexuality and relationship educators and certified sex therapists who have been working in the field of sexuality for more than two decades. They are the coauthors of the student workbook *Human Sexuality* (Prentice Hall, 1992) and the creators of Sex Ed Bingo (JLM Distributors, LLC). The Mirons team-teach a highly acclaimed college sex and relationships course at both The Community College of Baltimore County, Catonsville Campus, and Towson University. For the past decade, they have developed and run 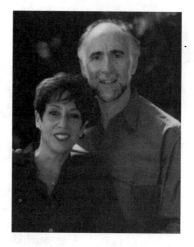 sexuality education retreats and workshops for parents and teens. The Mirons have appeared on numerous television and radio programs and their friendly faces have been found on the pages of many publications.

Charles Miron obtained his Ph.D. from the University of Maryland. He is a licensed clinical psychologist and coordinator of the psychology discipline at the Catonsville Campus of The Community College of Baltimore County. Amy Miron holds a master's degree in counseling from Johns Hopkins University and is a member of The Community College of Baltimore County and Towson University adjunct faculties. Happily married since 1967, they are the proud parents of two amazing adult daughters, Jill and Lynne.

Fast, Friendly, and Easy to Use
www.freespirit.com

Browse the catalog

Info & extras

Many ways to search

Quick check-out

Stop in and see!

Our Web site makes it easy to find the positive, reliable resources you need to empower teens and kids of all ages.

The Catalog.
Start browsing with just one click.

Beyond the Home Page.
Information and extras such as links and downloads.

The Search Box.
Find anything superfast.

Your Voice.
See testimonials from customers like you.

Request the Catalog.
Browse our catalog on paper, too!

The Nitty-Gritty.
Toll-free numbers, online ordering information, and more.

The 411.
News, reviews, awards, and special events.

Our Web site is a secure commerce site. All of the personal information you enter at our site—including your name, address, and credit card number—is secure. So you can order with confidence when you order online from Free Spirit!

For a fast and easy way to receive our practical tips, helpful information, and special offers, send your email address to upbeatnews@freespirit.com. View a sample letter and our privacy policy at *www.freespirit.com*.

1.800.735.7323 • fax 612.337.5050 • help4kids@freespirit.com